Emerging Issues in Family and Individual Resilience

Series Editors
Amanda W. Harrist
Oklahoma State University
Stillwater, OK, USA

Stephan M. Wilson
Oklahoma State University
Stillwater, OK, USA

Each year the Oklahoma State University's Center for Family Resilience holds a conference where distinguished and rising scholars from diverse disciplines discuss cutting-edge work and foster the community of educators and researchers in the field of family resilience. Presenting research-based knowledge from a range of academic disciplines such as family studies, human development, psychology, sociology, social work, education, law, and medicine, the series facilitates the development of evidence-based resilience practices, programs, and policies for those working with families at risk.

More information about this series at http://www.springer.com/series/13415

Jennifer L. Jones • Kami L. Gallus
Editors

Belonging and Resilience in Individuals with Developmental Disabilities

Community and Family Engagement

Springer

Editors
Jennifer L. Jones
Human Development and Family Science
Oklahoma State University
Stillwater, OK, USA

Kami L. Gallus
Human Development and Family Science
Oklahoma State University
Stillwater, OK, USA

ISSN 2366-6072 ISSN 2366-6080 (electronic)
Emerging Issues in Family and Individual Resilience
ISBN 978-3-030-81276-8 ISBN 978-3-030-81277-5 (eBook)
https://doi.org/10.1007/978-3-030-81277-5

This Springer imprint is published by the registered company Springer Nature Switzerland AG
The registered company address is: Gewerbestrasse 11, 6330 Cham, Switzerland

To our trailblazers: G, Michael, and Krista.

Preface

We wholeheartedly believe disability is a natural part of human diversity and when individuals with disabilities are embraced within their communities, everyone benefits. Ongoing efforts of parents, self-advocates, and professionals over the last several decades have focused on inclusion of individuals with intellectual and developmental disabilities (IDD: Wehmeyer, 2013). Significant work in research, policy, and practice (American Association on Intellectual and Developmental Disabilities, 2016) have led to positive changes in (special) education (e.g., segregated classrooms to inclusive education), employment (e.g., sheltered workshops to integrated employment), and living (e.g., institutionalization to community living). While these shifts forged the path to inclusion for some, many individuals with IDD and their families still remain on the fringes (Ali et al., 2012).

Since 2013, it has been an honor to focus our scholarship at Oklahoma State University on creating environments where everyone is seen, heard, and valued as full members within their families and communities. Built on the core belief that disability is a natural part of human diversity, we have equipped students, researchers, and practitioners to become agents of change alongside individuals and families. What began 8 years ago as a single research study quickly expanded to numerous research and community engagement projects that culminated in the opening of the Institute for Developmental Disabilities at Oklahoma State University. Each subsequent project within the Institute for Developmental Disabilities is united by a common theme: fostering resilient families and communities where individuals with IDD experience true belonging and an enhanced quality of life.

The current volume examines belonging as a key protective factor for enhancing resilience for individuals with IDD and their families. The development of this volume was inspired by leaders within the field of intellectual and developmental disabilities, many of whom so graciously agreed to speak at the OSU Center for Family Resilience's 2020 Chautauqua and subsequently author chapters in the current volume. In particular, Dr. Erik Carter's work on belonging (2016) resonated with and inspired much of our research and community engagement. Unbeknownst to him, Dr. Carter's work supported our ideas that relationships are key to improving lives and building resilient families and communities. We are grateful for the opportunity to explore how Dr. Carter's ten dimensions of belonging can be applied beyond faith communities to enhance resilience for all individuals, families, and communities.

Much to our delight, the seventh edition of the American Psychological Association Manual (APA: American Psychological Association, 2020) was released a few months after we began planning for the 2020 Chautauqua and writing the current volume. The current APA manual includes extensive revisions to bias-free language, including language and terms to use and those to avoid regarding disability. The manual provides principles that require authors to avoid perpetuating demeaning attitudes and guidelines for language that is affirming and inclusive. In compliance with the principles and guidelines regarding disability, the current volume uses person-first language emphasizing the person, not the individual's disabling condition, except in cases where an individual prefers identity-first language. We believe the evolving understanding of how language impacts our mental models leads to belonging and resilience. As such, we endorse the manual's instructions to avoid the use of bias-free language (including relevance of mentioning disability and avoiding negative and condescending terminology). We invite and strongly encourage readers to carefully review the manual's principles and guidelines.

The broad aim of the current volume centers on understanding IDD and resilience from systemic and social-ecological perspectives, emphasizing the roles of professionals, families, and communities in combating long-standing segregation and discrimination. At the heart of a systems orientation is an emphasis on relationships. As Bateson (1979) suggested, we believe this subtle, but powerful shift in our approach to working alongside individuals and families is generating a difference that makes a difference. By uncovering new information about the roles of family and community relationships, the current work strives to empower and enhance the lives of individuals often systematically excluded from full participation in their communities.

Our goal for the current volume is to explore belonging across diverse professional contexts and fields utilizing a person-centered approach that acknowledges the significant lifelong role of family members and emphasizes reflective practice for professionals. Chapters by leading experts address key issues across the lifespan and community contexts, including family-professional partnerships, universal design for learning, mental health, spirituality, research ethics and design, and future planning. In the chapters that follow, researchers and practitioners present innovative scholarship that fosters belonging and contributes to enhancing individual, family, and community resilience.

Stillwater, OK, USA

Jennifer L. Jones
Kami L. Gallus

References

Ali, A., Hassiotis, A., Strydom, A., & King, M. (2012). Self stigma in people with intellectual disabilities and courtesy stigma in family careers: A systematic review. *Research in Developmental Disabilities, 33*, 2122–2140. https://doi.org/10.1016/j.ridd.2012.06.013

American Association on Intellectual and Developmental Disabilities. (2016). *Critical issues in intellectual and developmental disabilities: Contemporary research, practice, and policy*. American Association on Intellectual and Developmental Disabilities.

American Psychological Association. (2020). *Publication manual of the American Psychological Association* (7th ed.). American Psychological Association. https://doi.org/10.1037/0000165-000

Bateson, G. (1979). *Mind and nature: A necessary unity* (Vol. 255). Bantam Books.

Carter, E. W. (2016). A place of belonging: Research at the intersection of faith and disability. *Review & Expositor, 113*(2), 167–180. https://doi.org/10.1177/0034637316637861

Wehmeyer, M. L. (Ed.). (2013). *The story of intellectual disability*. Paul H. Brookes.

Acknowledgments

We would like to thank the Department of Human Development and Family Science in the College of Education and Human Sciences at Oklahoma State University (OSU) for supporting the OSU Center for Family Resilience's 2020 Chautauqua, the conference that brought many outstanding scholars and practitioners together to focus on fostering belonging and resilience in individuals with developmental disabilities. Speakers – leading experts from diverse fields of study – addressed key issues across the lifespan and community contexts. Each speaker provided stimulating ideas that continue to influence conversations among the many key stakeholders, including family members, state developmental disabilities and provider agency personnel, academics, and practitioners in attendance across the 2-day event.

We also would like to express our gratitude to Dr. Michael Merten, former director and Dr. Amanda Harrist, associate director of OSU's Center for Family Resilience (CFR), for inviting us to organize the 11th Annual Chautauqua and for their ongoing support of this project. Throughout the planning process and our work together as colleagues, Drs. Merten and Harrist welcomed, accepted, and supported our big ideas. We also appreciate our fellow colleagues who graciously reviewed chapters and provided their feedback. Likewise, we extend our deep appreciation to John Giada with the Oklahoma Chapter of the American Association on Intellectual and Developmental Disabilities for the financial support of the 2020 Chautauqua. Last, but certainly not least, many thanks go to OSU graduate student, Tia Claybrook, for her gracious tolerance of our "impressive" attention to detail. In every sense of the word and in the true spirit of belonging, we needed Tia to pull this off and appreciate how she took care of every little detail.

Contents

About the Series Editors

Amanda W. Harrist received her Ph.D. in child and family studies from the University of Tennessee, Knoxville. She is currently a professor of human development and family science at Oklahoma State University, where she is also associate director for education and translation at the Center for Family Resilience and an administrative core director of human and community research training for the Center for Integrative Research on Childhood Adversity (CIRCA). Her research is focused on understanding psychosocial risk and protective processes in children's social contexts, particularly the parent-child relationship and peer relations at school.

Stephan M. Wilson is currently the dean of the College of Education and Human Sciences. He is a Ph.D. graduate in child and family studies from the University of Tennessee, Knoxville. He is an NCFR Fellow, Fulbright Fellow, Regents Professor at Oklahoma State University, and Legend recognition of the American Association of Family and Consumer Sciences, and has numerous teaching, research, and community engagement recognitions. His areas of expertise include cross-cultural family science and adolescent social competence.

About the Editors

Jennifer L. Jones is an associate professor of human development and family science and director of the Institute for Developmental Disabilities at Oklahoma State University. Dr. Jones received her Ph.D. in human development and family science from Oklahoma State University. Dr. Jones' deep respect and appreciation for individuals with intellectual and developmental disabilities and their families informs all aspects of her scholarship and is a driving force in her research, instruction, and community engagement. Her work in communities and in academia over the past 25 years have focused on improving the quality of life for individuals with intellectual and developmental disabilities and their families. Like many, Dr. Jones' passion and beliefs are deeply personal as a mother of a son with intellectual disability. Dr. Jones is grateful for the places of welcome and belonging she and her family have experienced and strives to create environments where people with and without disabilities can flourish together.

Kami L. Gallus is a professor at the Institute for Developmental Disabilities at Oklahoma State University. Dr. Gallus received her Ph.D. in marriage and family therapy from Texas Tech University. A licensed marriage and family therapist, Dr. Gallus' scholarship focuses on enhancing individual functioning, belonging, and relationship outcomes among vulnerable, often marginalized, and traditionally under-served populations, including female trauma survivors, at-risk youth, and individuals with intellectual and developmental disabilities. In contrast to a deficit model, which views vulnerability as a fixed internal trait, Dr. Gallus' scholarship conceptualizes vulnerability from a social ecological model, thus resulting from the person-environment fit. Ultimately, her systemic approach to applied research and clinical work focuses not on fixing or curing the individual, but rather on changing the understanding of the individual across contexts to provide supports that enhance the quality of life for all.

Contributors

Erik W. Carter Vanderbilt University, Nashville, TN, USA

Micah Fialka-Feldman Syracuse University, Syracuse, NY, USA

Kami L. Gallus Oklahoma State University, Stillwater, OK, USA

Bill Gaventa Institute on Theology and Disability, Austin, TX, USA

Karyn Harvey Park Ave Group, Baltimore, MD, USA

Jennifer L. Jones Oklahoma State University, Stillwater, OK, USA

Katherine McDonald Syracuse University, Syracuse, NY, USA

Loui Lord Nelson The UDL Approach, Indianapolis, IN, USA

Ariel Schwartz Boston University, Boston, MA, USA

Lynne T. Tomasa University of Arizona, Tucson, AZ, USA

Emily Tucker East Carolina University, Greenville, NC, USA

Ann Turnbull University of Kansas, Pittsboro, NC, USA

Rud Turnbull University of Kansas, Pittsboro, NC, USA

Heather J. Williamson Northern Arizona University, Flagstaff, AZ, USA

Chapter 1
Disability as Diversity: Rethinking Resilience for Individuals with Intellectual and Developmental Disabilities and Families

Jennifer L. Jones and Kami L. Gallus

Disability is a natural part of human diversity. With 15% of the global population experiencing a disability, individuals with disabilities make up the world's largest minority group (World Health Organization [WHO], 2019). Decades of research shows that when individuals with disabilities are embraced in communities, everyone benefits (Mahar et al., 2013; Mansell et al., 2002; Tucker et al., 2020). However, individuals with intellectual and developmental disabilities (IDD) and their families continue to encounter systemic and attitudinal barriers that perpetuate segregation and discrimination (Ali et al., 2012; Wehmeyer, 2013). Historically, individuals with IDD have been marginalized, and professional terminology has far too often been used to label and isolate individuals.

The current chapter begins with an overview of the terminology and diagnostic criteria associated with IDD. Next, we discuss the three waves of the disability movement, followed by the theoretical frameworks of the medical model and the social-ecological model and how these perspectives influence the lives of individuals and families. Finally, we introduce the construct of resilience and propose how creating and promoting belonging may serve as a key protective factor in fostering resilience among individuals with IDD and their families.

J. L. Jones (✉) · K. L. Gallus
Oklahoma State University, Stillwater, OK, USA
e-mail: jennifer.jones@okstate.edu

J. L. Jones, K. L. Gallus (eds.), *Belonging and Resilience in Individuals with Developmental Disabilities*, Emerging Issues in Family and Individual Resilience, https://doi.org/10.1007/978-3-030-81277-5_1

1.1 Intellectual and Developmental Disabilities

Disabilities can take many different forms including—but not limited to—hearing, vision, ambulatory, developmental, and intellectual (World Health Organization, 2019). Severe, persistent mental and/or physical developmental impairments are referred to as *developmental disabilities* (U.S. Department of Health and Human Services, 2000). This term includes an expansive group of conditions that impact a person's daily functioning. Developmental disabilities manifest before the age of 22 and are expected to last throughout life with significant limitations appearing in at least three of the following areas: self-care, receptive and expressive language, learning, mobility, self-direction, independent living, and/or money management. Some developmental disabilities may be primarily physical (e.g., epilepsy or blindness) or primarily cognitive (e.g., dyslexia). Others involve both physical and cognitive disabilities stemming from genetic or other causes, such as Down syndrome and fetal alcohol syndrome.

Intellectual disability is one of the most common developmental disabilities in the United States, with an estimated prevalence rate of approximately 1% of the population (American Psychiatric Association, 2013). The American Association on Intellectual and Developmental Disabilities (AAIDD) defines *intellectual disability* as originating before the age of 18 and characterized by significant limitations both in intellectual functioning (i.e., reasoning, learning, problem-solving) and in adaptive behavior, which covers a range of everyday social and practical skills (e.g., managing money, schedules, routines, social interactions; Schalock et al., 2010). Intellectual disability is a singular diagnostic term with multiple genetic (e.g., Down syndrome, Fragile X syndrome) and/or environmental (e.g., prenatal alcohol exposure, malnutrition) causes.

There have been significant shifts in the terminology used to describe the phenomenon now known as *intellectual disability*. Throughout the twentieth century, language shifted from *feeble-minded* to *mental retardation* with institutional classification systems of *idiot*, *moron*, or *imbecile* and educational categories of *educable* or *trainable* (Wehmeyer, 2013). At the turn of the twenty-first century, in an effort led by and with self-advocates (i.e., individuals with intellectual and developmental disabilities advocating for their own interests, desires, needs, and rights), the term *intellectual disability* replaced the term *mental retardation* in diagnostic manuals, service-delivery systems, and policies. This change in terminology is much more than an attempt at political correctness. The change reflects an understanding of disability that evolved from a person-centered trait (i.e., deficit) to a human phenomenon resulting from organic and social factors (Schalock, 2013). Since intellectual and developmental disabilities frequently co-occur and professionals often work with individuals who experience both, the terms are often combined to *intellectual and developmental disabilities* (Schalock et al., 2010).

1.2 Three Waves of the Disability Movement

The changes in terminology and diagnostic criteria have been heavily influenced by the disability movement (see Wehmeyer, 2013; Wehmeyer et al., 2000). Since the early 1900s, three waves of the movement (professional, parent, self-advocacy and self-determination) illustrate changes not only in language but also in the services available to and treatment of individuals and families. In our experience, these same three waves also serve to illustrate how most individuals and families are introduced to the language of IDD and learn to navigate two cultures: the mainstream culture of typical development and the subculture of intellectual and developmental disabilities. As with any movement, the disability movement includes individuals with direct personal experience (i.e., individuals, family members) and those who support and work alongside individuals with IDD.

1.2.1 Professionals

For the first half of the 1900s, professionals were viewed as the ultimate experts. Individuals with IDD were segregated from their families and society and placed in large state-run institutions where sterilization was practiced to control the spread of feeble-mindedness. Leaders and decision-makers in the field of IDD were often physicians who served as superintendents of the state institutions. Parents and society assumed professionals knew best, and individuals were not granted the most basic civil rights (Schalock & Wehmeyer, 2013).

While we often punctuate how the professional wave "ended" nearly 70 years ago, most parents today still begin their journey, seeking answers from professionals. Medical professionals often provide the first diagnosis, introducing parents to a new language. In our interviews with family members whose aging loved ones were transitioning out of state institutions—the only home many of these loved ones had ever known—we heard parent after parent share the emotion and memories of the first time they heard a professional use the language of disability to define their child (Jones & Gallus, 2016). For many of these family members, whose loved ones were 50, 60, and even 70 years old at the time of our interviews, neither the passage of time or the lifetime of ongoing involvement of professionals and systems of care seemed to dampen the emotion behind these memories. While the professional movement wave may have crested 70 years ago, professionals continue to play a critical role in the lives of individuals with IDD and their families.

1.2.2 Parents

With the return of many veterans with disabilities from World War II, a shift occurred, and the parent movement emerged in the early 1950s. People with disabilities were viewed as "objects to be fixed, cured, or rehabilitated, and simultaneously pitied" (Wehmeyer et al., 2000, p. 107). As parents began to advocate publicly for their children with disabilities, the *poster child* became a primary strategy in fundraising. Poster children promoted an understanding of individuals with IDD of all ages as innocent, eternal children. In contrast to the professional movement, when individuals with IDD were feared and families experienced social shame and blame, the parent movement promoted an understanding of individuals with disabilities as needing societal care, protection, and pity. While pity toward individuals with IDD does not lead to today's desirable outcomes of empowerment and inclusion, enhanced social awareness during this time period set the stage for many of today's leading disability organizations (e.g., The Arc, 2020; Special Olympics, 2020) that were born out of a parent or family member's advocacy. Professionals joined parents in developing services and lobbying for legislation to ensure basic civil rights for individuals with disabilities (Wehmeyer et al., 2000).

Today, parents of individuals with IDD face the unique circumstance of "lifespan parenting," the task of active caregiving from birth until either the parent's death or the death of the child. Although many parents report positive outcomes associated with their caregiving role, as with any life context, research also illustrates how the unique challenges associated with disability can negatively affect the well-being of families (Bayat, 2007; Burke et al., 2018). Even when individuals do not reside in the family home, caregiving is still a lifelong experience (Jones & Gallus, 2016). Long-term caregiving leads to various stressors and health disparities for parents of individuals with IDD, which often extend to siblings who may be enlisted to care for family members when parents are no longer able (Burke et al., 2018). Thus, while the time period of the parent movement from the 1950s to 1970s is often highlighted, research and experience demonstrate that parental involvement and advocacy are ongoing within the lives of individuals with IDD.

1.2.3 Self-Advocacy and Self-Determination

With the foundation of advocacy laid by parents, individuals with IDD began speaking for themselves, as the third wave, self-advocacy and self-determination, emerged during the 1970s and 1980s (Wehmeyer et al., 2000). Self-advocacy and self-determination were fueled by the normalization principle and the deinstitutionalization movement. The normalization principle refers to creating conditions where individuals with disability experience the normal respect extended to human beings leading to consideration of individual choices, desires, and aspirations (Nirje, 1969); whereas, the deinstitutionalization movement refers to changes in primary residence of individuals with IDD from institutions to living in the community with residential supports (Ferguson et al., 2013). Together, the normalization principle and deinstitutionalization have led to broader inclusion of individuals with disabilities in community life. Self-determination reflects the belief that all individuals have the right to make choices and direct their own lives and is a key dimension of individual quality of life (Schalock et al., 2005; Shogren, 2016). Self-advocates have spent the past 50 years fighting for the right to choose where they live and work and with whom they interact. Decades of research now show that self-determination is a key dimension of the quality of life and individuals with and without disabilities who are self-determined have more positive outcomes in education, employment, and relationships (Shogren, 2016). Professionals across diverse fields have the opportunity to come alongside self-advocates to further advance policies and practices that promote the health and well-being of individuals and their families.

1.3 Theoretical Perspectives

1.3.1 Shifting from the Medical Model to the Social-Ecological Model

To gain a better understanding of individuals with IDD, it is important to look beyond terminology and the historical movements to the underlying theoretical perspectives that influence social understanding and, subsequently, the experiences of individuals and families. The medical model is the dominant lens through which society broadly defines and understands disability. While the medical model served an important function, this model primarily views individuals in terms of deficit and classifies disability as a fixed trait residing permanently within the individual (Schalock et al., 2010). In contrast, social-ecological model of disability focuses not on fixing or curing the individual, but rather on changing our understanding of individuals within contexts to provide effective supports. Supports include resources and strategies that aim to promote the development, education, interests, and personal well-being of a person and that enhance individual functioning. From a social-ecological perspective, the disability does not lie within the person; rather it is the disparity between the demands of the environment and the person's current performance. The social-ecological model is not a denial or minimization of cognitive impairment; rather it places the emphasis on supports (Shogren, 2013). Table 1.1 illustrates differences in how the medical model and social-ecological model view disability.

The social-ecological model views disability as a multidimensional and fluid state of human functioning in relation to environmental demands (Schalock et al., 2010). Through this lens, an individual's support needs stem from five dimensions: intellectual abilities, adaptive behavior, health, participation, and context (see Conceptual Framework of Human Functioning in Schalock et al., 2010). The

Table 1.1 Medical model versus social-ecological model of disability

Medical model	Social-ecological model
Disability is a fixed trait residing within the individual	Disability is a fluid state of functioning
Disabled people are broken or abnormal and should be fixed, cured, and/or prevented	Disability is a natural part of human diversity, and supports help enhance individual and family outcomes
Disabled people need caregivers and professionals to make decisions for them. They are an object of charity and receiver of help	Individuals should be supported to live the life of their own choosing supported by their families and communities

social-ecological perspective assumes that individuals experience barriers not as a direct result of their disability, but rather as a result of the lack of environmental supports (Shogren, 2013). *Supports* include "resources and strategies that aim to promote the development, education, interests, and personal well-being of a person and that enhance individual functioning" (Schalock et al., 2010, p. 18). Individuals with IDD are not inherently different from individuals without IDD—all human functioning is enhanced through supports (e.g., many use the GPS technology on our smart phones). *Thoughtful planning of and access to* individualized supports is needed for individuals to carry out daily activities, meet their long-term goals, and realize their dreams.

A social-ecological understanding of *disability as diversity* shifts our focus from increasing personal competence to understanding and providing the supports individuals need across a variety of environments. As a result, supports cannot be "prescribed" solely from a fixed diagnostic label. The nature and extent of supports needed to participate in family and community life are ever evolving. Support needs are highly individualized (as the saying goes, "if you have met *one* person with autism, you have met *one* person with autism"), fluid, continuous, and ever-changing across time and context.

1.3.2 Resilience Framework

Similar to the disability field, the conceptualization of resilience has been influenced by the medical model, with initial research focused on personal competence. Early models emerging from the positive psychology movement (Seligman & Csikszentmihalyi, 2000) viewed resilience as an individual trait determined by one's long-term ability to respond to adversity in a healthy and adaptive manner. Masten et al. (1990) defined resilience as "the process of, capacity for, or outcome of successful adaptation despite challenging or threatening circumstances" (p. 426). As a result, models of individual resilience often viewed disability as adversity and defined resilience as one's ability to overcome or thrive *in spite of the presence of a disabling condition.* In some of the early models of resilience, disabilities were an assumed tragedy, and parents and siblings were seen as heroic for thriving in spite of having a family member with a disability (Dykens, 2005). Similar to the social-ecological perspective, more recent conceptualizations of resilience and research from systemic and contextual lenses highlight that individuals do not exist—or thrive—in isolation. From a broader systems view, resilience goes beyond an individual characteristic to a dynamic interaction between individuals and their environments (Masten & Wright, 2010).

1.3.2.1 Resilience and Families

With a majority of individuals receiving support for daily living from a family caregiver (Larson et al., 2018), family relationships play a uniquely important role in promoting resilience among individuals with IDD and their families. Families of individuals with IDD experience unique challenges across the lifespan (see Fujiura, 2010; Given et al., 2013; Heller et al., 2015; Hewitt et al., 2013). While some families function well (Bayat, 2007), research also illustrates how these unique challenges can negatively affect the health and well-being of some families (Brown et al., 2003; Greenberg et al., 1993; Jokinen & Brown, 2011). Research also indicates that access to social support and promoting adaptation to meet everyday challenges help families mitigate many of the negative effects, often noted as outcomes in family research (Caldwell et al., 2018; Jones & Gallus, 2016; McConnell & Savage, 2015). Because family members are the largest providers of care for individuals with IDD in the United States, it is imperative that families are adequately supported. Despite the acknowledgment of the importance of family supports, there is much work to be done in defining and identifying best practices and policy for effectively supporting families (Burke et al., 2018; Hewitt et al., 2013). Ongoing work is necessary to enhance understanding and knowledge of what helps families navigate significant transitions and risks throughout the lifespan (Caldwell et al., 2018).

Consolidating individual and family resilience literature, Henry et al. (2015) conceptualized the family resilience model (FRM), providing a promising framework for understanding the processes leading to resilience in families. Based on the integration of ideas from family systems theory, family stress theory, and individual resilience (Hawley & DeHaan, 1996), the FRM is a strengths-based approach to understanding family adaptation to significant risk (Henry et al., 2015; see Fig. 1.1). Within the FRM, significant risks are inherently value neutral. Risks can arise from any event that disrupts ongoing family dynamics (e.g., roles, rules, rituals) and impacts family functioning (Harrist et al., 2018; Henry et al., 2015; Patterson, 2002). Whether an event is labeled as positive or negative by the family or society is irrelevant to the activation of the family resilience processes. As a strengths-based and systemic model, the FRM holds potential to explain what helps individuals and their family members navigate and positively adapt to a lifetime of individual and systemic challenges and changes.

Henry et al. (2015) suggest families experience both vulnerabilities and protections expressed at multiple levels, including individual functioning, dyadic

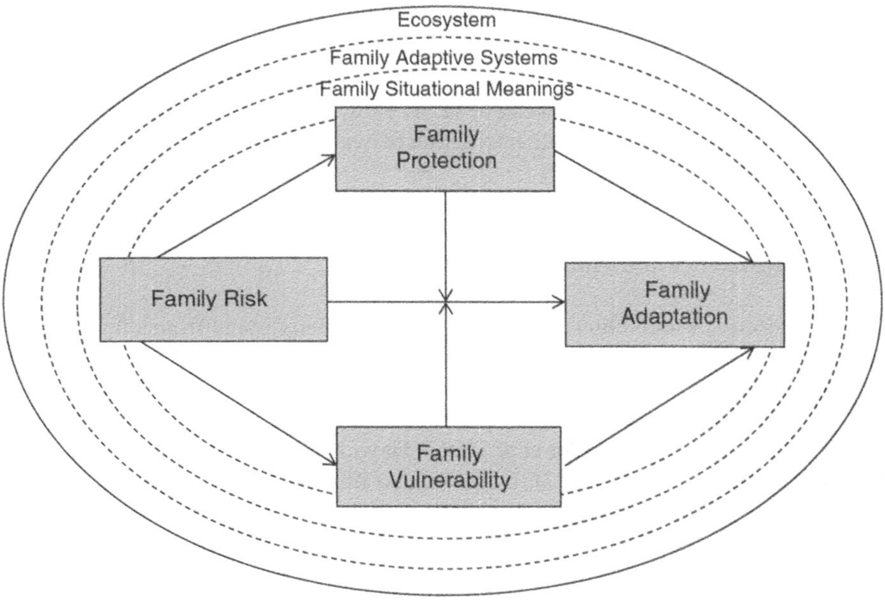

Fig. 1.1 Family resilience model (FRM)
Note: Reprinted from "Family resilience: Moving into the third wave" by Carolyn S. Henry, Amanda S. Morris, and Amanda W. Harrist, **2015**, Family Relations, 64(**1**), p. **31**. Copyright **2015** by the National Council on Family Relations. Reprinted with permission

relationships, and the overall social system. Within the FRM, resilience emerges in the family through adaptive processes, such as family meaning-making, rhythm, and communication. Integrated together, these multidimensional components and complex processes represent a family's ability to adapt and thus achieve resilience. Yet, as further noted within the FRM, key resilience relationships extend beyond the family into the community. The interrelatedness of families and communities is particularly relevant for individuals with IDD who rely heavily on social systems for services and supports. Efforts to enhance resilience must actively engage communities and social environments in which resilience can be nurtured.

1.3.2.2 Belonging: A Key to Resilience

Ultimately, the multidimensional and dynamic process of resilience requires wholehearted engagement with—not withdrawal from or denial of—the realities of life. When we view disability through the social-ecological model, it is the environmental and societal barriers that are most problematic for individuals with IDD and their families, not the differences in how one's brain or body works. The desire to be included by your community, to have meaningful work, and to share life with people you love and who love you—to *belong*—are not "special needs"; they are very ordinary needs. When individuals feel valued, needed, respected, and significant, a true sense of belonging occurs (Mahar et al., 2013).

Using a family resilience perspective to understand the lives of individuals with IDD and their families expands the focus beyond inclusion and individualized supports to identifying and mobilizing family and community strengths that foster positive growth and adaptation. Conceptually, *belonging* may serve as a key protective factor particularly relevant in facilitating resilience among individuals with IDD and their families (see Carter, 2016; this volume, Chap. 2). Initial research within the field of IDD has explored belonging as a multidimensional process within the context of faith communities (Carter, 2016). As the proceeding chapters outline, belonging is an important process that can be fostered within and across all contexts of resilience—individual, family, and community.

Questions for Thought and Discussion

1. How have the three waves of the disability movement impacted individual, family, and community resilience?
2. What model of disability has framed your understanding of intellectual and developmental disability?
3. How does the social-ecological framework provide a lens for understanding disability as diversity?
4. How might understanding disability as diversity in your scholarship or practice lead to belonging and resilience for individuals and families?

References

Ali, A., Hassiotis, A., Strydom, A., & King, M. (2012). Self stigma in people with intellectual disabilities and courtesy stigma in family carers: A systematic review. *Research in Developmental Disabilities, 33*, 2122–2140. https://doi.org/10.1016/j.ridd.2012.06.013.

American Psychiatric Association. (2013). *Diagnostic and statistical manual of mental disorders (DSM-5®)*. American Psychiatric Association.

Bayat, M. (2007). Evidence of resilience in families of children with autism. *Journal of Intellectual Disability Research, 51*(9), 702–714. https://doi.org/10.1111/j.1365-2788.2007.00960.x.

Brown, I., Anand, S., Alan-Fung, W. L., Isaacs, B., & Baum, N. (2003). Family quality of life: Canadian results from an international study. *Journal of Developmental and Physical Disabilities, 15*, 207–229. https://doi.org/10.1023/A:1024931022773.

Burke, M. M., Lulinski, A., Jones, J. L., & Gallus, K. L. (2018). A review of supports and services for adults with intellectual and developmental disabilities (IDD) and their families in the United States: Past and present contexts impacting future research, practice and policy. In M. Burke (Series Ed.), *International review of research in developmental disabilities: Volume 54. Service delivery systems for individuals with intellectual and developmental disabilities and their families across the lifespan* (pp. 137–176). https://doi.org/10.1016/bs.irrdd.2018.07.005.

Caldwell, J. A., Jones, J. L., Gallus, K. L., & Henry, C. S. (2018). Empowerment and resilience in families of adults with intellectual and developmental disabilities. *Intellectual and Developmental Disabilities, 56*(5), 374–388. https://doi.org/10.1352/1934-9556-56.5.374.

Carter, E. W. (2016). A place of belonging: Research at the intersection of faith and disability. *Review & Expositor, 113*(2), 167–180. https://doi.org/10.1177/0034637316637861.

Dykens, E. M. (2005). Happiness, well-being, and character strengths: Outcomes for families and siblings of persons with mental retardation. *Mental Retardation, 43*, 360–364. https://doi.org/10.1352/0047-6765(2005)43[360:HWACSO]2.0.CO;2.

Ferguson, D. L., Ferguson, P. M., & Wehmeyer, M. L. (2013). The self-advocacy movement. In M. L. Wehmeyer (Ed.), *The story of intellectual disability* (pp. 233–276). Paul H. Brookes.

Fujiura, G. T. (2010). Aging families and the demographics of family financial support of adults with disabilities. *Journal of Disability Policy Studies, 20*(4), 241–250. https://doi.org/10.1177/1044207309350560.

Given, C. W., Given, B. A., Sherwood, P., & DeVoss, D. (2013). Early adult caregivers: Characteristics, challenges, and intervention approaches. In R. C. Talley & R. J. V. Montgomery (Eds.), *Caregiving across the lifespan* (pp. 81–103). Springer.

Greenberg, J. S., Seltzer, M. M., & Greenley, J. R. (1993). Aging parents of adults with disabilities: The gratifications and frustrations of later-life caregiving. *The Gerontologist, 33*, 542–550. https://doi.org/10.1093/geront/33.4.542.

Harrist, A. W., Henry, C. S., Liu, C., & Morris, A. S. (2018). Family resilience: The power of rituals and routines in family adaptive systems. In B. Fiese (Ed.), *The APA handbook of contemporary family psychology, Volume 1: Foundations, methods, and changing forms* (pp. 223–239). American Psychological Association Press.

Hawley, D. R., & DeHaan, L. (1996). Toward a definition of family resilience: Integrating lifespan and family perspectives. *Family Process, 35*, 283–298. https://doi.org/10.1111/j.1545-5300.1996.00283.x.

Heller, T., Gibbons, H. M., & Fisher, D. (2015). Caregiving and family support interventions: Crossing networks of aging and developmental disabilities. *Intellectual and Developmental Disabilities, 53*(5), 329–345. https://doi.org/10.1352/1934-9556-53.5.329.

Henry, C. S., Morris, A. S., & Harrist, A. W. (2015). Family resilience: Moving into the third wave. *Family Relations, 64*(1), 22–43. https://doi.org/10.1111/fare.12106.

Hewitt, A., Agosta, J., Heller, T., Williams, A. C., & Reinke, J. (2013). Families of individuals with intellectual and developmental disabilities: Policy, funding, services, and experiences. *Intellectual and Developmental Disabilities, 51*(5), 349–359. https://doi.org/10.1352/1934-9556.51.5.349.

Jokinen, N. S., & Brown, R. I. (2011). Family quality of life and older-aged families of adults with an intellectual disability. In R. Kober (Ed.), *Enhancing the quality of life of people with intellectual disabilities: From theory to practice* (pp. 279–303). Springer.

Jones, J. L., & Gallus, K. L. (2016). Understanding deinstitutionalization: What families value and desire in the transition to community living. *Research and Practice for Persons with Severe Disabilities, 41*(2), 116–131. https://doi.org/10.1177/1540796916637050.

Larson, S. A., Eschenbacher, H. J., Anderson, L. L., Taylor, B., Pettingell, S., Hewitt, A., Sowers, M., & Bourne, M. L. (2018). *In-home and residential long-term supports and services for persons with intellectual or developmental disabilities: Status and trends through 2016.* University of Minnesota, Research and Training Center on Community Living, Institute on Community Integration.

Mahar, A. L., Cobigo, V., & Stuart, H. (2013). Conceptualizing belonging. *Disability and Rehabilitation, 35*(12), 1026–1032. https://doi.org/10.3109/09638288.2012.717584.

Mansell, J., Elliott, T., Beadle-Brown, J., Ashman, B., & Macdonald, S. (2002). Engagement in meaningful activity and "active support" of people with intellectual disabilities in residential care. *Research in Developmental Disabilities, 23*(5), 342–352. https://doi.org/10.1016/S0891-4222(02)00135-X.

Masten, A. S., & Wright, M. O. (2010). *Resilience over the lifespan: Developmental perspectives on resistance, recovery, and transformation* (pp. 213–237). Guilford.

Masten, A. S., Best, K. M., & Garmezy, N. (1990). Resilience and development. *Development and Psychopathology, 2*, 425–444. https://doi.org/10.1017/S0954579400005812.

McConnell, D., & Savage, A. (2015). Stress and resilience among families caring for children with intellectual disability: Expanding the research agenda. *Current Developmental Disorders Reports, 2*, 100–109. https://doi.org/10.1007/s40474-015-0040-z.

Nirje, B. (1969). The normalization principle and its human management implications. In R. B. Kugel & W. Wolfensberger (Eds.), *Changing residential patterns for the mentally retarded* (pp. 363–376). President's Committee on Mental Retardation.

Patterson, J. M. (2002). Understanding family resilience. *Journal of Clinical Psychology, 58*(3), 233–246. https://doi.org/10.1002/jclp.10019.

Schalock, R. L. (2013). Introduction to the intellectual disability construct. In M. L. Wehmeyer (Ed.), *The story of intellectual disability* (pp. 1–15). Paul H. Brookes.

Schalock, R. L., & Wehmeyer, M. (2013). The parent movement: Late modern times "1950ce – 1980ce". In M. L. Wehmeyer (Ed.), *The story of intellectual disability* (pp. 187–232). Paul H. Brookes.

Schalock, R. L., Verdugo, M. A., Jenaro, C., Wang, M., Wehmeyer, M., Jiancheng, X., & Lachapelle, Y. (2005). Cross-cultural study of quality of life indicators. *American Journal on Mental Retardation, 110*(4), 298–311. https://doi.org/10.1352/0895-8017(2005)110[298:CSOQOL]2.0.CO;2.

Schalock, R. L., Borthwick-Duffy, S. A., Bradley, V. J., Buntinx, W. H. E., Coulter, D. L., Craig, E. M., Gomez, S. C., Lachapelle, Y., Luckasson, R., Reeve, A., Shogren, K. A., Snell, M. E., Spreat, S., Tasse', M. J., Thompson, J. R., Verdugo-Alonso, M. A., Wehmeyer, M. L., & Yeager, M. H. (2010). *Intellectual disability: Definition, classification and systems of supports* (11th ed.). American Association on Intellectual and Developmental Disabilities.

Seligman, M. E. P., & Csikszentmihalyi, M. (2000). Positive psychology: An introduction. *American Psychologist, 55*(1), 5–14. https://doi.org/10.1037/0003-066X.55.1.5.

Shogren, K. A. (2013). Positive psychology and disability: A historical analysis. In M. L. Wehmeyer (Ed.), *The Oxford handbook of positive psychology and disability* (pp. 19–33). Oxford University Press.

Shogren, K. A. (2016). Self-determination and self-advocacy. In *Critical issues in intellectual and developmental disabilities: Contemporary research, practice, and policy* (pp. 1–18). American Association on Intellectual and Developmental Disabilities.

Special Olympics. (2020). *History.* http://www.specialolympics.org/Sections/What_We_Do/History_of_Special_Olympics.aspx.

The Arc. (2020). *Who we are.* http://www.thearc.org/who-we-are.

Tucker, E. C., Jones, J. L., Gallus, K. L., Emerson, S. R., & Manning-Ouellette, A. L. (2020). *Let's Take A Walk*: Exploring intellectual disability as diversity in higher education. *Journal of College and Character, 21*(3), 157–170. https://doi.org/10.1080/2194587X.2020.1781659.

U.S. Department of Health and Human Services. (2000). *Developmental disabilities assistance and Bill of Rights Act amendments of 2000*, PL 106-402, 45 CFR 1385.3-Definitions.

Wehmeyer, M. L. (Ed.). (2013). *The story of intellectual disability*. Paul H. Brookes.

Wehmeyer, M., Bersani, H. J., & Gagne, R. (2000). Riding the third wave: Self-determination and self-advocacy in the 21st century. *Focus on Autism and Other Developmental Disabilities, 15*, 106–115. https://doi.org/10.1177/108835760001500206.

World Health Organization. (2019). *World report on disability.* https://www.who.int/disabilities/world_report/2011/report/en/.

Chapter 2
Dimensions of Belonging for Individuals with Intellectual and Developmental Disabilities

Erik W. Carter

We flourish most in the midst of community. This reflects an increasingly common refrain across many different disciplines. Public health researchers point to the strong association between having vibrant social connections and experiencing good physical and mental health (Leigh-Hunt et al., 2017). Social scientists cite the myriad ways in which supportive relationships contribute to overall well-being (Chu et al., 2010). Educational scholars emphasize the strong associations among positive peer relationships, school climate, and student learning outcomes (Wentzel, 2017). Theologians declare that we were created for community and formed for friendship with our neighbors (Swinton, 2012). To say it simply, it is not good to be alone.

Many aspects of thriving are shaped by the relationships, supports, and experiences available within the communities of which individuals with intellectual and developmental disabilities (IDD) are part (e.g., Boehm & Carter, 2016; Zuna et al., 2010). Indeed, a healthy community can provide a place of companionship, enjoyment, assistance, encouragement, meaning, and participation for all members. Yet connections to community life have historically been restricted for individuals with IDD. Whether the setting is a school, workplace, neighborhood, religious congregation, or other community program, most studies find that individuals with IDD participate substantially less often than others or in more limited ways than they would like (e.g., National Core Indicators, 2019; National Organization on Disability, 2010; Newman et al., 2011). Although some individuals with disabilities enjoy inclusion and belonging, many more experience only the peripheries of community life.

E. W. Carter (✉)
Vanderbilt University, Nashville, TN, USA
e-mail: erik.carter@vanderbilt.du

J. L. Jones, K. L. Gallus (eds.), *Belonging and Resilience in Individuals with Developmental Disabilities*, Emerging Issues in Family and Individual Resilience, https://doi.org/10.1007/978-3-030-81277-5_2

The purpose of this chapter is to address the place of belonging within our collective efforts to promote the flourishing of individuals with IDD and their families. I begin with an overview of how our pursuits within the field of disability have evolved over time and are pushing us to think beyond mere location. Next, I present a framework for reflecting upon and fostering belonging within an inclusive community. I then offer implications for practice and policy aimed at promoting the inclusion and belonging of individuals with disabilities. I conclude with recommendations for future resilience-oriented research that could enhance our understanding of belonging and the factors that shape it.

2.1 Our Evolving Aims

The last century has been a period of substantial progress in the opportunities and supports available to individuals with IDD and their families (Agran et al., 2014; Wehmeyer, 2013). Indeed, the experiences we have pursued for—and more recently with—individuals with disabilities and their families have changed quite dramatically. Throughout so much of human history, individuals with IDD were *excluded* from most aspects of community life. They were denied involvement in local schools, workplaces, neighborhoods, and other available activities; they were missing from the membership rolls of most communities. In response to this widespread isolation, early advocacy often focused on creating new spaces for individuals with IDD to learn, work, live, and recreate. But these opportunities were usually provided within specialized settings that essentially kept people with disabilities *segregated* from anyone else who did not have a similar label. Separate special education schools, sheltered workshops, and residential institutions were established across the country and around the world. In most communities, everyday life excluded people with disabilities.

2.1.1 Integration as a Goal

As legislation, policy, and research advanced, the landscape continued to change (Wehmeyer, 2013). The focus of many fields shifted toward ensuring individuals with IDD were *integrated* within ordinary aspects of community life. Access to neighborhood schools, area businesses, local congregations, and other community programs expanded considerably. Yet within each of these settings, the prevailing support models for individuals with disabilities involved the creation of experiences that were largely distinct from the experiences of their peers without disabilities. Self-contained classrooms, employment enclaves, special needs ministries, group homes, and specialized recreation programs all placed individuals with IDD near, but not really among, their peers without disabilities. Life was experienced adjacent to—rather than in the company of—one another.

2.1.2 Inclusion as a Goal

The current emphasis within the field is on ensuring individuals with IDD are *included* fully within the life of any community (Agran et al., 2014). New approaches to service delivery emphasize supporting individuals within the same classrooms, clubs, jobs, congregational activities, and community groups as anyone else. By supporting shared activities in ordinary settings, individuals with and without disabilities have regular opportunities to meet one another and spend time together. Although inclusion has yet to take hold in widespread ways, it is clear that relationships still do not develop automatically for individuals with IDD simply from spending time in the midst of others (Biggs & Carter, 2017). Something more may be needed if shared spaces are to lead to shared lives.

2.1.3 Beyond Integration and Inclusion

Figure 2.1 illustrates these four portraits of community for individuals with IDD—*exclusion*, *segregation*, *integration*, and *inclusion*. Although recent history certainly leans toward integration and inclusion, it is important to emphasize that all four depictions can still be observed in contemporary society. Indeed, they can often stand side-by-side within and across cities, states, and countries—much like a living history museum of service delivery models across the decades. More importantly, there is a growing sense that none of these four portraits depicts the final destination of this evolving movement. People want to be more than merely integrated or included within a community; they want to experience real *belonging* within that community (Carter, 2016; Hall, 2010; Swinton, 2012). Like anyone else, individuals with IDD say they want to belong (Carter et al., 2016a; Fulford & Cobigo, 2016; Hall, 2010).

What, then, does it mean to truly belong within a community? How can we know whether individuals with IDD experience belonging in the ways and places that matter most to them? How might this experience of belonging contribute to their

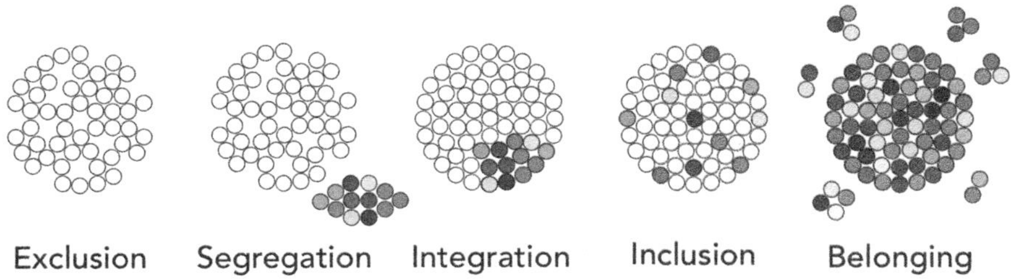

Fig. 2.1 Five portraits of communities in relation to individuals with intellectual and developmental disabilities

resilience and thriving? These are just a few of the crucial questions for organizations, agencies, and programs charged with promoting the flourishing of individuals with disabilities and their families.

2.2 Dimensions of Belonging

Belonging has been conceptualized in varied ways across diverse fields (e.g., Allen & Bowles, 2012; Hagerty et al., 1992; Mahar et al., 2013). Framed broadly, it refers to the assurance of acceptance and value within a particular group. Belonging is often described as having elements of intimacy, connectedness, membership, commitment, solidarity, or reciprocity. Moreover, it is presumed to be a universal need that cuts across cultures, people, and time (Baumeister & Leary, 1995; Maslow, 1954). We all need to belong—somewhere and to someone. Surprisingly, this construct has received scant attention within the disability literature (e.g., Carter et al., 2016a; McConkey et al., 2019; Schnorr, 1990; Schroeder et al., 2021; Smith et al., 2015; Strnadová et al., 2018). For a group of individuals most at risk for isolation and exclusion, belonging may require more careful consideration and intentional investment.

In this section, I address ten dimensions of belonging that may have particular salience to individuals with IDD, as well as their families. In doing so, I draw upon research addressing the inclusion, relationships, and belonging of individuals with IDD across school, work, congregational, and other community contexts. Although belonging is not often addressed explicitly in the literature, the postures and practices that may contribute to belonging have been a long-standing focus of empirical research. Within the following framework, belonging is experienced when people are *present*, *invited*, *welcomed*, *known*, *accepted*, *supported*, *heard*, *befriended*, *needed*, and *loved* (see Fig. 2.2). Each of these dimensions is described in the following sections.

2.2.1 To Be Present

Conversations about integration and inclusion often emphasize location—the extent to which individuals with disability are present in the same places available to others without disabilities in a particular community. Similarly, presence is critical to belonging. There is an important spatial aspect to belonging; in other words, location matters. Schools, workplaces, congregations, and local communities are all comprised of activities, routines, events, and rituals around which their members periodically or regularly come together. It is within and through these encounters that relationships are forged, supports are exchanged, and affiliations are strengthened.

Reflection Questions	What are we already doing well?	What could we do better or differently?	What should we start doing next?
Present Is our community comprised of individuals with and without IDD?			
Invited Are we pursuing their presence and actively extending new invitations?			
Welcomed Are we extending a warm welcome whenever they arrive?			
Known Do we know them personally and for the strengths they possess?			
Accepted Are we receiving them unconditionally and graciously?			
Heard Are we seeking out their preferences and perspectives on issues that matter?			
Supported Are we providing the assistance they need to participate fully and meaningfully?			
Befriended Are we creating opportunities for friendships to form and deepen?			
Needed Are we recognizing and receiving their talents, gifts, and contributions?			
Loved Are we loving them deeply and unconditionally?			

Fig. 2.2 Tool to help communities reflect on the belonging of individuals and their families
Note. Adapted from E. W. Carter, "Dimensions of Belonging: Listening to and Learning from Families." Presentation at the 40th annual TASH Conference, Portland, Oregon, 2015

Yet *absence* is still more common than *presence* for many individuals with IDD. Consider just a few of the contexts in which people typically spend their time. In the United States, school-age children without disabilities attend their neighborhood school and take an array of interesting classes alongside a wide range of peers. In contrast, almost half (49%) of students with intellectual disability spend the majority of their day in a self-contained classroom apart from peers without disabilities, and 7% attend a different school altogether (U.S. Department of Education, 2017). Nearly half (41%) of all Americans continue their education after high school by attending college or some other type of postsecondary training program (U.S. Department of Education, 2020). Yet few young adults with intellectual disability are present on these college campuses within 4 years of high school graduation (Newman et al., 2009). Moreover, less than 5% of all higher education institutions in the United States have launched formal programs to support the enrollment of students with intellectual disability (Grigal & Papay, 2018). Nearly three-quarters of working-age Americans are contributing their time and talents in businesses throughout their communities (Bureau of Labor Statistics, 2020). Less than one fifth (20%) of adults with intellectual disability are present in these same workplaces (Winsor et al., 2018).

Across these and so many other areas, persistent participation gaps exist between people with and without IDD (National Organization on Disability, 2010). More importantly, there are sizable gaps between the types of involvement people with disabilities say they want and their actual participation in those same experiences (Carter, 2015). For example, more than half of youth with intellectual disability want to pursue postsecondary education, and more than 90% want a paid job in the community (Lipscomb et al., 2017). Such absence separates people from most other dimensions of belonging by limiting the extent to which someone can be known, accepted, heard, befriended, needed, and loved. Fostering belonging begins by supporting the presence of individuals with disabilities within the places and among the people that matter most to them. Inclusion provides the foundation for belonging, but does not ensure it. After all, it is so very hard to belong where you are never or rarely present.

For individuals and organizations committed to fostering belonging for individuals with disabilities, ongoing and careful reflection is needed on the barriers that stand in the way of presence. Barriers to inclusion still abound in most communities. Some reside in the accessibility, awareness, attitudes, and practices of communities; others are evident in the expectations, supports, resources, and priorities of service systems (Agran et al., 2014; Carter et al., 2017). This constellation of barriers must be removed as the foundation for belonging (i.e., presence) is laid.

2.2.2 *To Be Invited*

The pathway to presence often requires extending new invitations. As a community notices that individuals with disabilities and their families are not yet in their midst, community members may begin reaching out to encourage involvement. This usually takes the form of announcements—broad notifications about community offerings and, perhaps, their desire to be inclusive of individuals with disabilities.

For example, schools might distribute information about their extracurricular offerings, congregations about their worship services and children's ministries, recreation programs about their upcoming events, and companies about their desire for a diverse workforce. But such general announcements can still leave uncertainty among individuals with IDD and their families. Amidst a history of prior exclusion or inhospitable encounters, new proclamations of a warm reception may be viewed with reservations or doubts. The possibility that they may be the one exception to the pronouncement that "all are welcome" still lingers for many people.

Invitations can help counter this concern. Personal requests to attend an event or join a group can assure someone that his or her presence is actually desired. Indeed, attendance may be more likely to follow an invitation than an announcement. But invitations are not merely a remedy to absence. Invitations also communicate something important about the value of a person from the perspective of the community. They assure people that they are wanted and perhaps even needed. This shift from passively awaiting someone's potential arrival to actively pursuing their presence can be influential in fostering a sense of belonging. A person's presence does not catch the community by surprise when actively sought out.

The motivation to extend new invitations can emerge from different directions. Some communities realize they are missing out on the talents, strengths, and gifts that individuals with disabilities might offer (Lindsay et al., 2018; Tucker et al., 2020). Others realize the absence of individuals with disabilities conflicts with the core mission of their community. For example, most religious traditions have position statements or theological beliefs that affirm the inclusion of people with disabilities (Carter, 2021). Similarly, many schools have mission statements that accentuate "every child" or affirm that "all means all." Some community groups are formally charged with serving all corners of their communities without distinction. And more and more workplaces are actively striving to better reflect the diversity of their local community. Sadly, invitations to individuals with IDD are still surprisingly rare. Few educators, employers, congregations, and community groups are actively and vigorously pursuing the presence of individuals with disabilities and their families.

2.2.3 *To Be Welcomed*

Early encounters can impact the extent to which people experience belonging within a particular community. Among individuals with IDD and their families, stories about their community experiences often include themes of unexpected welcoming or deep wounding. The former response encourages guests to enter further, while the latter response persuades them to turn away. Although awareness of and attitudes toward people with disabilities have improved substantially in recent decades, the tenor of a community's initial response is still hard to predict in advance (Scior & Werner, 2015). Some community members still feel reluctant or resistant; others are hesitant or even hostile. Each of these unwelcoming postures nearly always translates into avoidance.

In contrast, belonging is nurtured when individuals with disabilities and their families encounter generous hospitality within a community. The response of the community to their presence is one of delight, friendliness, courtesy, and authenticity. Parents have described this response as being welcomed without condition, warmly embraced, treated like family, or feeling at home (Carter et al., 2016a). The avenues through which welcome is communicated tend to involve ordinary gestures much more than extraordinary actions. For example, hospitality involves greeting people personally, remembering their names, drawing them into conversation, asking about their week, encouraging their participation, anticipating their needs, inviting them to other events, and noticing when they are absent and reaching out to find out why. These everyday actions communicate to people that they are wanted and welcomed. In other words, welcoming individuals with disabilities and their families is not substantially different from welcoming anyone else. However, it requires intentionality and an ongoing commitment.

For communities that do not have a history of including people with IDD, uncertainty may exist about how best to move forward in this area. They may benefit from receiving guidance on how to engage with individuals who may communicate differently, require ongoing assistance, or behave in unfamiliar ways; how to talk about disability in respectful and relevant ways; or how to design their programs and spaces with their entire community in mind. Such efforts can ensure that educators, employers, co-workers, greeters, and other community members are comfortable and confident in their interactions *before* someone arrives to their communities for the first time. Disability organizations can be instrumental in these efforts by providing training to schools, workplaces, and community programs on how to widen their welcome. For example, the *Inclusion Network of Nashville* offers workshops for arts, athletic, entertainment, educational, and government organizations on designing their activities and programs in ways that will be accessible and feel welcoming to individuals with disabilities. This has led to an array of new sensory friendly events and facility renovations.

2.2.4 To Be Known

Belonging is personal. The extent to which someone is known well by others in a community can impact their sense of connectedness and membership. To be noticed, recognized, and acknowledged by others are each important aspects of belonging (Schnorr, 1990; van Alphen et al., 2009). Yet individuals with disabilities are often overlooked, even when involved in inclusive activities. For example, observational studies in inclusive classrooms have found that some students with intellectual disability or autism still go the entire class periods without their peers initiating any conversations (Carter et al., 2008; Chung et al., 2012). Likewise, studies addressing integrated neighborhoods and workplaces find that some individuals with IDD still feel anonymous or ignored in the midst of others (Lysaght et al., 2012; Overmars-Marx et al., 2014). The transition from stranger to friend is a crucial marker of belonging.

How someone is known also makes a difference. Disability is so often discussed using the language of deficits and weaknesses (Wehmeyer, 2013). Indeed, most diagnostic labels and special education categories emphasize what someone cannot or struggles to do, ignoring their many talents and positive qualities. As a result, individuals with disabilities are often viewed throughout society primarily through the lens of limitations. They are known by their labels rather than by their names—seen for their weaknesses rather than for their strengths. Such labeling can serve to limit the experience of belonging because it presents an inaccurate or incomplete portrait of who a person is. Moreover, it deters communities from pursuing the presence of people with disabilities.

Communities committed to belonging adopt a very different perspective. They approach individuals with disabilities as *individuals*—each unique and worthy of getting to know personally and deeply. They seek to learn each person's story, and they strive to understand the interests, passions, skills, gifts, and talents the person brings to the community. As communities come to know each person well, they are better positioned to support, befriend, need, and love each person well. This strengths-based stance is consistent with how many family members describe their children or siblings with IDD (Carter et al., 2014, 2015, 2020). While affirming that individuals with IDD can possess enviable qualities (e.g., kindness, optimism, courage, empathy, gratitude, joy), valuable skills, and wide-ranging abilities, these studies also report that no two people possess the very same set of strengths and positive traits. Such findings suggest that disability organizations and agencies must come to know the strengths of each person they support and communicate those strengths in winsome ways to the communities the person is interested in joining.

2.2.5 To Be Accepted

It is one thing to be included; it is another to be accepted. Hundreds of studies have examined attitudes toward individuals with intellectual disability, autism, and other developmental disabilities within the general public and among various professionals (see reviews by Pelleboer-Gunnink et al., 2017, 2019; Scior, 2011). Overall, the awareness of people with IDD, accurate knowledge about disability and its impact, and views toward people with disabilities have improved over the last 50 years. These improvements have been driven by changes in service delivery models, greater visibility in the community, and public awareness campaigns. At the same time, stigma, stereotypes, and prejudice still persist in nearly every corner of contemporary society (Siperstein et al., 2007). Such views can substantially limit the extent to which individuals with IDD are invited and welcomed into the life of a community. Moreover, the persistence of negative attitudes undergird views around the world that individuals with intellectual disability should be served primarily in separate or specialized settings (Siperstein et al., 2003; Scior & Werner, 2015).

Belonging entails the assurance of acceptance. Whether in a school, workplace, congregation, neighborhood, or other social group, the affirmation that you are accepted as you are—without condition or caveat—is central to belonging. Acceptance feels quite different from mere tolerance. Shifting the attitudes of others, however, can be challenging work. The literature highlights several ways in which communities can be primed toward greater acceptance of individuals with disabilities. Formal awareness events or campaigns are sometimes used to increase understanding and acceptance of people with disabilities. For example, some schools, companies, and community groups host activities in conjunction with awareness months or days focused on developmental disabilities (March), Down syndrome (March 21 and October), cerebral palsy (March), autism (April), disability employment (October), and inclusive schools (first week of December). More targeted approaches include embedding curricular units within school courses or religious education programs, offering presentations or workshops, or disseminating informational materials (e.g., brochures, videos). The impact of these interventions has been promising (Leigers & Myers, 2015; Lindsay & Edwards, 2013), but information sharing alone is not sufficient. Personal contact is among the most powerful ways of promoting acceptance. In other words, genuine acceptance usually emerges from coming to know someone personally rather than from learning about someone abstractly. Indeed, research on attitude change suggests that promoting positive interactions over time may be the most effective way of changing views toward persons with disabilities (Scior & Werner, 2015; Tucker et al., 2020). It is in the midst of relationships that preconceived ideas about a person most likely may be overturned.

2.2.6 To Be Supported

Like anyone else, individuals with IDD will need support to participate meaningfully in the breadth of activities and routines that comprise a particular community. The difference is that this support must usually be more individualized, intensive, and intentional (Thompson et al., 2014). It is the absence of adequate and personalized support that limits the extent to which individuals with disabilities and their families can access the communities that matter most to them. The availability of needed assistance, adaptations, equipment, encouragement, facilitation, finances, information, instruction, modifications, materials, technology, or transportation often is inconsistent or limited. Providing the right support at the right time enables involvement in the experiences and relationships that make people feel like they belong. Moreover, this investment communicates to a person that his or her presence is truly desired. For families, access to supports can also be instrumental in helping them to navigate the expected and unanticipated stressors and challenges of life (Henry et al., 2015).

Research suggests that the form of support matters immensely. For example, schools, employment programs, and residential programs often employ individually assigned staff (e.g., paraprofessionals, job coaches, direct support providers) to deliver one-to-one support to individuals with IDD in general education classrooms, integrated workplaces, and community activities (Giangreco, 2010). However, this heavy reliance on specialized persons can inadvertently limit shared activities and stifle social connections within inclusive settings. In the absence of artful facilitation and planned fading, the ongoing presence of a third party can be stigmatizing or introduce an unnecessary mediator of interactions (Carter, 2018). In contrast, drawing upon natural supports (i.e., the people and resources that already exist within a place) whenever possible is strongly advocated. This might take the form of help from friends, co-workers, or fellow members; use of ubiquitous technologies (e.g., smart devices); access to existing processes or routines; and receipt of ordinary forms of available assistance (e.g., mentoring, financial assistance, transportation). For example, peer-mediated interventions are regularly used to support students with IDD in inclusive elementary, secondary, and postsecondary classrooms and campuses (Carter, 2017; Carter et al., 2019). Natural supports help forge connections with individuals who are part of the same community in lieu of (or in addition to) recruiting outside assistance. For families, these natural supports can provide some constancy amidst the uncertainty of service systems (Boehm & Carter, 2016).

Designing these supports requires careful planning. The combination of supports that will be most helpful for one person will look quite different for another. Likewise, supports should be matched to the demands of the different settings in which they participate. Person-centered planning can help discern an individual's preferences and priorities for support (Claes et al., 2010). Asking good questions is the best way to learn which types and timing of support will be most important. A variety of planning approaches have been advocated for use in schools, workplaces, congregations, and community settings (Carter et al., 2016b; Giangreco et al., 2011). Communities may also need guidance or training on how to deliver these supports and communicate their availability. However, communities committed to belonging for individuals with IDD see the provision of this support as essential rather than as an imposition.

2.2.7 *To Be Heard*

The perspectives of individuals with IDD have not often been sought. Throughout so much of the history of disability, the voices of professionals and parents have dominated the dialog (Agran et al., 2014). In recent decades, however, a shift toward self-advocacy has taken hold. Best practices now emphasize ensuring individuals with disability have a say in all aspects of their own lives (Wehmeyer et al., 2017). Being part of a community that also yearns to hear your voice can contribute to an assurance of belonging. To be heard, to have a seat at the table, to be listened to, to be acknowledged, to be asked what you think, or to have an influence—all communicate to people that their involvement and insights matter. Such phrases reflect the shift from being present to having a presence—from silence to salience. Being part of a community in which others seek out your input can be empowering and suggests that your presence makes a real difference.

Individuals with IDD may benefit from opportunities to learn and practice the skills needed to share their preferences and perspectives with others. The better people understand themselves (e.g., strengths, needs, interests, goals) and know their communities, the better positioned they will be to advocate for themselves and for others. Providing instruction in the areas of self-determination, assertiveness, advocacy, and leadership can also help individuals with IDD share their thoughts more effectively with others (Wehmeyer et al., 2017). For individuals with complex communication challenges or more significant cognitive impairments, it is important to identify augmentative and alternate communication (AAC) systems that can enable their voices to be heard (Biggs et al., 2018).

At the same time, communities may need to reflect on the formal and informal avenues through which they seek out the perspectives of their members. Where advisory councils, organizational boards, and leadership roles, and other committees exist, individuals with disabilities should be provided encouragement and supports to participate (Caldwell et al., 2009). When perspectives are sought on issues within the community, individuals with IDD should not be overlooked. Likewise, when advice or an opinion is needed, individuals with and without disabilities should readily turn to each other. Families and disability organizations can play a role in helping communities recognize the value in soliciting these overlooked perspectives and the importance of overcoming preconceived ideas about whose voice matters most.

2.2.8 *To Be Befriended*

Belonging is experienced best through relationships. People thrive most when in the company of others who know, need, and care about them. Having someone to talk with, walk with, cheer with, cry with, lunch with, lounge with, pray with, or play with can be a powerful antidote to loneliness and isolation. Unfortunately, many children and adults with IDD have very few relationships outside of their family members or the professionals involved in their lives (Simplican et al., 2015). Although loneliness and isolation are felt by many in the general population (Leigh-Hunt et al., 2017), the issue is more acute for individuals with disabilities. For example, more than one fifth (22%) of adults with IDD receiving public services and supports report having no friends who are not family members or paid staff (National Core Indicators, 2019). Among high school students, only 42% of youth with intellectual disability and 29% of youth with autism get together with friends at least once a week (Lipscomb et al., 2017). Interventions, treatments, services, and programs can do many good things for individuals with IDD, but they are rarely the pathway to belonging. Instead, it is the formation of friendships and other caring relationships that are most critical.

This dimension of belonging benefits from facilitation more than from force. Friendships do not emerge through mandate, legislation, or obligation; they cannot be declared or demanded. As Reinders (2011) notes:

> …being loved and befriended does something for you that rights and choice cannot possibly do. It brings you the invaluable experience of being chosen by someone else. Whatever it is that rights and choice can do—and we do not have to proof that they can do a lot of very important things—but whatever rights and choice can do, they are not going to make me your friend. (p. 433)

Although there is no guaranteed friendship formula, much can be said about the conditions under which individuals with IDD are most likely to get picked as friends (Amado, 2013; Biggs & Carter, 2017). These include providing people with access to ordinary experiences, ensuring they have reliable ways of communicating with others, connecting them with people who hold some interests in common, giving them valued roles within activities, preparing peers with relevant information (e.g., strengths, needs, and preferences of the person; ideas for supporting them effectively), and providing everyone with just enough support. Put simply, friendships are more likely to emerge when people participate in shared activities over time with others with whom they have shared connection. Sadly, prevailing practices substantially limit the extent to which individuals with IDD can access these important encounters with others. Inclusive practices can provide a rich context for friendship formation, but relationships are never automatic.

2.2.9 To Be Needed

People know they belong when they are needed by others. So much of the research on inclusive practices emphasizes the ways in which individuals with IDD might benefit from participating in the same activities as anyone else in their community. For example, studies examining inclusion within typical classrooms, workplaces, congregations, and neighborhoods have examined its positive impact on the skills, knowledge, interactions, relationships, health, and self-perceptions of individuals with disabilities (see reviews by Almalky, 2020; Carter, 2021; Chowdhury & Benson, 2011; Hagiwara et al., 2019). But the larger community also benefits from the presence and participation of individuals with disabilities (e.g., Lindsay et al., 2018; Peltier, 1997; Travers & Carter, 2021). When talents, gifts, abilities, and contributions are recognized and received by a community, people feel valued. Experiencing this reciprocity firsthand is an important aspect of belonging.

When individuals with IDD assume valued roles within a community, the ways in which they are viewed by others can begin to change (Wolfensberger, 1983). This might come from volunteering, taking on leadership responsibilities in a classroom or project, helping others in need in their community, participating in high-status activities, serving through one's faith community (e.g., greeter, usher, choir, altar server), having a meaningful job, assisting on important projects, having a role on a team, or contributing in any number of other ways. This shift from recipient to contributor brings a sense of significance and importance. Others in the community come to see you as integral, perhaps even as indispensable. As Swinton (2012) notes, "People need to be concerned when you are not there; your communities need to feel empty when you are not there. The world needs to be perceived as radically different when you are not there. Only when your absence stimulates feelings of emptiness will you know that you truly belong" (p. 183).

2.2.10 To Be Loved

Healthy communities are marked by love and wholehearted care for one another. This love can take many different forms—an affectionate regard, a deep concern, or an unconditional commitment. People tend to go to great lengths for those whom they love—they make allowances, they go the extra mile, they extend grace, they sacrifice their own interests, they avoid what is expedient, they work for another's good, and they offer forgiveness. Moreover, love leads people to care about someone's flourishing throughout all 7 days of the week—after school dismisses, outside of the workday, and beyond the benediction. When people talk about the communities that matter most to them, they often talk about the love they encounter there (Carter et al., 2016a; Strnadová et al., 2018). Where love abounds, belonging is much more likely to be experienced.

Yet how rarely love is mentioned in the professional literature. Love is not listed among our evidence-based interventions. It is never referenced in state or federal policies. It is avoided in discussions of everyday procedures and practices. It is never touched on in trainings. Such silence should not be interpreted as irrelevance. Love is central to belonging. As Reinders (2011) notes:

> Being loved by someone is what matters most in our lives. What we do not often think about, however, is the logic of this statement, and this logic is what I ask you to contemplate for a moment. *If 'being loved' is the most important thing in our lives, then the most important thing is something we cannot do by ourselves or on our own.* It is not a goal we can strive for, it is not something we can achieve. To be loved by someone implies that the most important thing in our lives is something we can only receive as a gift. (p. 432)

Perhaps the greatest of these ten dimensions of belonging is to be loved.

2.3 Implications for Practice

Belonging is profoundly important, but often elusive. What steps can communities take to become places in which individuals with IDD and their families are invited, present, welcomed, known, accepted, supported, heard, befriended, needed, and loved? First, this framework of belonging provides a helpful structure to guide reflection and identify relevant responses. Although the salience of belonging is likely to be endorsed in most communities, the postures and practices that lead toward it can be more difficult to articulate. The unpacking of this construct allows communities to consider each of the ten dimensions individually at a level that is actionable: What are we doing really well right now in each of these areas? What should we be doing better or differently? What next steps should we take in each area to strengthen our community? Figure 2.2 displays a reflection tool for guiding this discussion (Forest & Pearpoint, 1997). Inviting a cross-section of community members—including individuals with IDD and their families—to contribute to this reflection can ensure that multiple perspectives are heard.

Second, disability agencies and organizations committed to the flourishing of individuals with IDD should also consider whether the services and supports they deliver are leading toward belonging. In response to legislation, policy, and research calling for more inclusive approaches, many programs are in the midst of converting their service delivery models—from sheltered workshops to integrated employment, from self-contained classrooms to general education access, from congregate facilities to supported living, and from special needs ministries to universally designed worship (Agran et al., 2014). But this appeal to push beyond inclusion introduces a new focus and goal for agencies and organizations. Belonging emphasizes the primacy of relationships right alongside full participation. A classroom cannot be considered inclusive if no one talks to the student. A job cannot be called integrated employment if no one knows her name. And a new home cannot be described as community living if there are no neighbors embracing her. Figure 2.1 could provide a catalyst for discussions among program leadership: Which of these portraits best reflects our current service delivery model? What would it take to move in the direction of belonging? In addition, across the ten dimensions of belonging, presence is the only dimension consistently tracked within the field (e.g., percentage of people who are served in integrated employment, time spent in regular classrooms, number served in public and private institutions). What might it look like for organizations and agencies to document the other nine dimensions? How might it lead them to refine or reinvent their services if any dimensions were discovered to be absent?

Third, many communities will need to be persuaded or encouraged to move in this direction; others will need guidance on how to proceed further. This still represents new terrain for most schools, workplaces, congregations, and community programs in the United States and around the world (Agran et al., 2020; Braddock et al., 2017; Carter, 2021; Winsor et al., 2018). Disability organizations, agencies, and advocates will need to be winsome and wise as they call upon communities to widen their welcome. They should develop strong partnerships and commit to supporting others in these areas. Likewise, communities will need guidance on how best to move forward in many of the ten dimensions. Disability groups can share their experience and insights on removing barriers to participation, reaching out to the individuals they serve, creating hospitable spaces, seeing people's strengths, promoting awareness, providing meaningful supports, listening to new voices, facilitating relationships, and encouraging everyone's contributions. By offering information, assistance, training, encouragement, and accountability, these groups can help equip communities to respond differently to the presence of individuals with IDD in their midst.

2.4 Implications for Research and the Study of Resilience

The topic of belonging is beginning to receive more attention within the field of IDD. But research in this area is still in its infancy. Future studies are needed to examine a number of key questions related to this familiar—yet understudied—concept.

First, what does it mean to belong within a community? As is true with prominent constructs like inclusion (Ryndak et al., 2000), self-determination (Vicente et al., 2018), quality of life (Schalock et al., 2002), and community participation (Milner & Kelly, 2009), belonging may be prone to misunderstanding or misapplication. It is common to observe situations described using these different constructs that seem quite antithetical to their actual meaning. At present, there is no consensus definition of belonging within the field of disability. Moreover, the few available studies on this topic arrive at somewhat different conceptualizations of this construct (e.g., Carter et al., 2016a; Renwick et al., 2019; Schroeder et al., 2021; Strnadová et al., 2018). Additional research should explore how individuals with disabilities and their families interpret and experience belonging within the various communities they consider to be most important personally. Although the ten dimensions of belonging outlined in this chapter seem to have broad relevance, other dimensions and definitions are likely to emerge.

Second, how do we know whether individuals with IDD are experiencing belonging? The assessment of belonging is fraught with measurement challenges. Like other important concepts in the field (e.g., social inclusion, self-advocacy), belonging is multidimensional, personal, and contextual. In other words, it can mean somewhat different things to different people in different places at different times. With input from multiple stakeholders, it may be helpful to develop measures that can be used to examine belonging across different types of communities (e.g., schools, workplaces, congregations, communities) and different size groups. This collection of measures should include both observable and subjective indicators of belonging. Moreover, we need ways of understanding the experience of belonging among individuals who cannot speak or who have significant cognitive impairments. What behavioral or other indicators could serve as potential markers? For example, indicators related to each of the ten dimensions addressed in this chapter could be developed, applied, and validated across populations and settings.

Third, how might belonging contribute to flourishing and resilience in other areas of a person's life? When individuals with disabilities have valued roles within caring communities, the good things of life are expected to become available to them (Wolfensberger, 1983). The experience of belonging within a community provides access to relationships, supports, and opportunities that could enrich someone's life in myriad ways. To date, the connections between belonging and flourishing have yet to be examined empirically. There will undoubtedly be moderators and mediators. In addition, the pathways from one to the other should be explored in future studies.

Fourth, what are the risks associated with pursuing belonging as a distinct—and perhaps higher—outcome? Belonging is certainly not an entirely new aim within the field of disability. Even a cursory review of our history suggests that rejection can be as likely a response as embrace. Are there unanticipated consequences of shifting our accent from inclusion to belonging? For communities that step into this space, conflict and contention are likely to emerge as they expand who they invite and revisit how they gather (Simplican, 2019). What are the tensions that communities experience as they make these movements? How might those challenges be negotiated and resolved in ways that are mutually beneficial? And what might be the roles of self-advocates, families, disability organizations, and others in guiding these conversations?

2.5 Summary

Over the last few decades, the inclusion of individuals with IDD has advanced in nearly every aspect of community life—schools, workplaces, religious communities, neighborhoods, and many others. Although the considerable progress being made around the world is worth celebrating, there is a destination that lies beyond inclusion that should be vigorously pursued. Like anyone else, individuals with disabilities want to experience belonging. To be present, invited, welcomed, known, accepted, supported, heard, befriended, needed, and loved—each of these ten dimensions of belonging contributes to the assurance of one's value and place within a meaningful community. What might we do to equip communities across the country to adopt new postures and practices in each of these areas? How might communities become stronger and richer by making this investment? And what difference will it make in the lives of people with and without disabilities?

Questions for Thought and Discussion

1. What is the next step for building belonging for individuals with intellectual and developmental disabilities in your scholarship or practice?
2. What would look different in the communities you are part of if individuals with intellectual and developmental disabilities were truly invited, present, welcomed, known, accepted, supported, cared for, befriended, needed, and loved?
3. How does one's sense of true belonging impact individual, family, and community resilience?

References

Agran, M., Brown, F., Hughes, C., Quirk, C., & Ryndak, D. (Eds.). (2014). *Equity and full participation for individuals with severe disabilities: A vision for the future*. Brookes.

Agran, M., Jackson, L., Kurth, J. A., Ryndak, D., Burnette, K., Jameson, M., Zagona, A., Fitzpatrick, H., & Wehmeyer, M. L. (2020). Why aren't students with severe disabilities being placed in general education classrooms: Examining the relations among classroom placement, learner outcomes, and other factors. *Research and Practice for Persons with Severe Disabilities, 45*(1), 4–13. https://doi.org/10.1177/1540796919878134.

Allen, K. A., & Bowles, T. (2012). Belonging as a guiding principle in the education of adolescents. *Australian Journal of Educational & Developmental Psychology, 12*, 108–119. https://files.eric.ed.gov/fulltext/EJ1002251.pdf.

Almalky, H. A. (2020). Employment outcomes for individuals with intellectual and developmental disabilities: A literature review. *Children and Youth Services Review, 109*, 1–10. https://doi.org/10.1016/j.childyouth.2019.104656.

Amado, A. N. (2013). *Friends: Connecting people with disabilities and community members*. University of Minnesota, Institute on Community Integration.

Baumeister, R. F., & Leary, M. R. (1995). The need to belong: Desire for interpersonal attachments as a fundamental human motivation. *Psychological Bulletin, 117*(3), 497–529. https://doi.org/10.1037/0033-2909.117.3.497.

Biggs, E. E., & Carter, E. W. (2017). Supporting the social lives of students with intellectual disability. In M. L. Wehmeyer & K. A. Shogren (Eds.), *Handbook of research-based practices for educating students with intellectual disability* (pp. 235–254). Routledge.

Biggs, E. E., Carter, E. W., & Gilson, C. B. (2018). Systematic review of interventions involving aided AAC modeling for children with complex communication needs. *American Journal on Intellectual and Developmental Disabilities, 123*(5), 443–473. https://doi.org/10.1352/1944-7558-123.5.443.

Boehm, T. L., & Carter, E. W. (2016). Systematic review of informal relationships among parents of individuals with intellectual disability or autism. *Research and Practice for Persons with Severe Disabilities, 41*(3), 173–190. https://doi.org/10.1177/1540796916657339.

Braddock, D., Hemp, R., Tanis, E. S., Wu, J., & Haffer, L. (2017). *The state of the states in intellectual and developmental disabilities: 2017*. American Association on Intellectual and Developmental Disabilities.

Bureau of Labor Statistics. (2020). *Employment situation new release: February 2020*. Author.

Caldwell, J., Hauss, S., & Stark, B. (2009). Participation of individuals with developmental disabilities and families on advisory boards and committees. *Journal of Disability Policy Studies, 20*(2), 101–109. https://doi.org/10.1177/1044207308327744.

Carter, E. W. (2015). What matters most: Toward a future of flourishing. *TASH Connections, 41*(3), 10–20. https://www.gvsu.edu/autismcenter/start-connecting-what-matters-most-toward-a-future-341.htm.

Carter, E. W. (2016). A place of belonging: Research at the intersection of faith and disability. *Review & Expositor, 113*(2), 167–180. https://doi.org/10.1177/0034637316637861.

Carter, E. W. (2017). The promise and practice of peer support arrangements for students with intellectual and developmental disabilities. *International Review of Research in Developmental Disabilities, 52*, 141–174. https://doi.org/10.1016/bs.irrdd.2017.04.001.

Carter, E. W. (2018). Supporting the social lives of secondary students with severe disabilities: Critical elements for effective intervention. *Journal of Emotional and Behavioral Disorders, 26*(1), 52–61. https://doi.org/10.1177/1063426617739253.

Carter, E. W. (2021). Spirituality and supports for individuals with intellectual and developmental disabilities and their families. In L. M. Glidden, L. Abbeduto, L. L. McIntyre, & M. J. Tassé (Eds.), *APA handbook on intellectual and developmental disabilities* (pp. 419–442). American Psychological Association.

Carter, E. W. (2021). Research on disability and congregational inclusion: What we know and where we might go. *Journal of Religion and Disability*.
Carter, E. W., Biggs, E. E., & Boehm, T. L. (2016a). Being present versus having a presence: Dimensions of belonging for young people with disabilities and their families. *Christian Education Journal, 13*(1), 127–146. https://doi.org/10.1177/073989131601300109.
Carter, E. W., Boehm, T. L., Biggs, E. E., Annandale, N. H., Taylor, C., Logeman, A. K., & Liu, R. Y. (2015). Known for my strengths: Positive traits of transition-age youth with intellectual disability or autism. *Research and Practice for Persons with Severe Disabilities, 40*(2), 101–119. https://doi.org/10.1177/1540796915592158.
Carter, E. W., Brock, M. E., & Trainor, A. A. (2014). Transition assessment and planning for youth with severe intellectual and developmental disabilities. *The Journal of Special Education, 47*(4), 245–255. https://doi.org/10.1177/0022466912456241.
Carter, E. W., Carlton, M. B., & Travers, H. (2020). Seeing strengths: Young adults and their siblings with intellectual and developmental disabilities. *Journal of Applied Research in Intellectual Disabilities, 33*(3), 574–583. https://doi.org/10.1111/jar.12701.
Carter, E. W., Endress, T., Gustafson, J., Shouse, J., Taylor, C., Utley, A., Amado, A., Nord, D., Timmons, J., Kleinert, H., Tyree, M., Canevaro, A., Seay, P., Gaventa, W., & Allen, W. (2016b). *Putting faith to work: A guide for congregations and communities on connecting job seekers with disabilities to meaningful work*. Collaborative on Faith and Disability.
Carter, E. W., Gustafson, J. R., Mackay, M. M., Martin, K., Parlsey, M., Graves, J., Day, T., McCabe, L., Lazarz, H., McMillan, E., Beeson, T., Schiro-Geist, C., Williams, M., & Cayton, J. (2019). Motivations and expectations of peer mentors within inclusive higher education programs for students with intellectual disability. *Career Development and Transition for Exceptional Individuals, 42*(3), 168–178. https://doi.org/10.1177/2165143418779989.
Carter, E. W., McMillan, E., Willis, W., & Partnership, T. W. (2017). The TennesseeWorks Partnership: Elevating employment outcomes for people with intellectual and developmental disabilities. *Journal of Vocational Rehabilitation, 47*(3), 365–378. https://doi.org/10.3233/JVR-170909.
Carter, E. W., Sisco, L. G., Brown, L., Brickham, D., & Al-Khabbaz, Z. A. (2008). Peer interactions and academic engagement of youth with developmental disabilities in inclusive middle and high school classrooms. *American Journal on Mental Retardation, 113*(6), 479–494. https://doi.org/10.1352/2008.113:479-494.
Chowdhury, M., & Benson, B. A. (2011). Deinstitutionalization and quality of life of individuals with intellectual disability: A review of the international literature. *Journal of Policy and Practice in Intellectual Disabilities, 8*(4), 256–265. https://doi.org/10.1111/j.1741-1130.2011.00325.x.
Chu, P. S., Saucier, D. A., & Hafner, E. (2010). Meta-analysis of the relationships between social support and well-being in children and adolescents. *Journal of Social and Clinical Psychology, 29*(6), 624–645. https://doi.org/10.1521/jscp.2010.29.6.624.
Chung, Y., Carter, E. W., & Sisco, L. G. (2012). Social interaction of students with severe disabilities who use augmentative and alternative communication in inclusive classrooms. *American Journal on Intellectual and Developmental Disabilities, 117*(5), 349–367. https://doi.org/10.1352/1944-7558-117.5.349.
Claes, C., Van Hove, G., Vandevelde, S., van Loon, J., & Shalock, R. L. (2010). Person-centered planning: Analysis of research and effectiveness. *Intellectual and Developmental Disabilities, 48*(6), 432–453. https://doi.org/10.1352/1934-9556-48.6.432.
Forest, M., & Pearpoint, J. (1997). *Four easy questions*. Inclusion Press.
Fulford, C., & Cobigo, V. (2016). Friendships and intimate relationships among people with intellectual disabilities: A thematic synthesis. *Journal of Applied Research in Intellectual Disabilities, 31*(1), 98–105. https://doi.org/10.1111/jar.12312.
Giangreco, M. F. (2010). One-to-one paraprofessionals for students with disabilities in inclusive classrooms: Is conventional wisdom wrong? *Intellectual and Developmental Disabilities, 48*(1), 1–13. https://doi.org/10.1352/1934-9556-48.1.1.

Giangreco, M. F., Cloninger, C. J., & Iverson, V. S. (2011). *Choosing options and accommodations for children (COACH): A guide to educational planning for students with disabilities* (3rd ed.). Brookes.

Grigal, M., & Papay, C. (2018). The promise of postsecondary education for students with intellectual disability. *New Directions for Adult & Continuing Education, 2018*(160), 77–88. https://doi.org/10.1002/ace.20301.

Hall, E. (2010). Spaces of social inclusion and belonging for people with intellectual disabilities. *Journal of Intellectual Disability Research, 54*(s1), 48–57. https://doi.org/10.1111/j.1365-2788.2009.01237.x.

Hagerty, B. M. K., Lynch-Sauer, J., Patusky, K. L., Bouwsema, M., & Collier, P. (1992). Sense of belonging: A vital mental health concept. *Archives of Psychiatric Nursing, 6*(3), 172–177. https://doi.org/10.1016/0883-9417(92)90028-H.

Hagiwara, H., Amor, A. M., Shogren, K. A., Thompson, J. R., Verdugo, M. A., Burke, K. M., Uyanik, H., & Aguayo, V. (2019). International trends in inclusive education intervention research: A literature review. *Education and Training in Autism and Developmental Disabilities, 54*(1), 3–17. https://eric.ed.gov/?id=EJ1205734.

Henry, C. S., Morris, A. S., & Harrist, A. W. (2015). Family resilience: Moving into the third wave. *Family Relations, 64*(1), 22–43. https://doi.org/10.1111/fare.12106.

Leigers, K. L., & Myers, C. T. (2015). Effect of duration of peer awareness education on attitudes toward students with disabilities: A systematic review. *Journal of Occupational Therapy, Schools, & Early Intervention, 8*(1), 79–96. https://doi.org/10.1080/19411243.2015.1021067.

Leigh-Hunt, N., Bagguley, D., Bash, K., Turner, V., Turnbull, S., Valtorta, N., & Cann, W. (2017). An overview of systematic reviews on the public health consequences of social isolation and loneliness. *Public Health, 152*, 157–171. https://doi.org/10.1016/j.puhe.2017.07.035.

Lindsay, S., Cagliostro, E., Albarico, M., Mortaji, N., & Karon, L. (2018). A systematic review of the benefits of hiring people with disabilities. *Journal of Occupational Rehabilitation, 28*(4), 634–655. https://doi.org/10.1007/s10926-018-9756-z.

Lindsay, S., & Edwards, A. (2013). A systematic review of disability awareness interventions for children and youth. *Disability and Rehabilitation, 35*(8), 623–646. https://doi.org/10.3109/09638288.2012.702850.

Lipscomb, S., Haimson, J., Liu, A. Y., Burghardt, J., Johnson, D. R., & Thurlow, M. L. (2017). *Preparing for life after high school: The characteristics and experiences of youth in special education* (Vol. Vol. 2). U.S. Department of Education.

Lysaght, R., Cobigo, V., & Hamilton, K. (2012). Inclusion as a focus of employment-related research in intellectual disability from 2000 to 2010: A scoping review. *Disability and Rehabilitation, 16*(16), 1339–1350. https://doi.org/10.3109/09638288.2011.644023.

Mahar, A. L., Cobigo, V., & Stuart, H. (2013). Conceptualizing belonging. *Disability and Rehabilitation, 35*(12), 1026–1032. https://doi.org/10.3109/09638288.2012.717584.

Maslow, A. (1954). *Motivation and personality*. Harpers.

McConkey, R., Peng, C., Merritt, M., & Shellard, A. (2019). The meaning of social inclusion to players with and without intellectual disability in Unified Sports teams. *Inclusion, 7*(4), 234–243. https://doi.org/10.1352/2326-6988-7.4.234.

Milner, P., & Kelly, M. (2009). Community participation and inclusion: People with disabilities defining their place. *Disability & Society, 24*(1), 47–62. https://doi.org/10.1080/09687590802535410.

National Core Indicators. (2019). *In-person survey: 2017–18 final report*. https://www.nationalcoreindicators.org.

National Organization on Disability. (2010). *Kessler Foundation/NOD survey of Americans with disabilities*. Author.

Newman, L., Wagner, M., Cameto, R., & Knokey, A. M. (2009). *The post-high school outcomes of youth with disabilities up to 4 years after high school*. SRI International.

Newman, L., Wagner, M., Knokey, A. M., Marder, C., Nagle, K., Shaver, D., & Wei, X. (2011). *The post-high school outcomes of young adults with disabilities up to 8 years after high school.* SRI International.

Overmars-Marx, T., Thomese, F., Verdonschot, M., & Meininger, H. (2014). Advancing social inclusion in the neighbourhood for people with an intellectual disability: An exploration of the literature. *Disability & Society, 29*(2), 255–274. https://doi.org/10.1080/09687599.2013.800469.

Pelleboer-Gunnink, H. A., van Oorsouw, W. M. W. J., van Weeghel, J., & Embregts, P. J. C. M. (2017). Mainstream health professionals' stigmatising attitudes towards people with intellectual disabilities: A systematic review. *Journal of Intellectual Disability Research, 61*(5), 411–434. https://doi.org/10.1111/jir.12353.

Pelleboer-Gunnink, H. A., van Oorsouw, W. M. W. J., van Weeghel, J., & Embregts, P. J. C. M. (2019). Stigma research in the field of intellectual disabilities: A scoping review on the perspective of care providers. *International Journal of Developmental Disabilities*. https://doi.org/10.1080/20473869.2019.1616990.

Peltier, G. L. (1997). The effect of inclusion on non-disabled children: A review of the research. *Contemporary Education, 68*(4), 234–238. https://eric.ed.gov/?id=EJ556298.

Reinders, H. S. (2011). The power of inclusion and friendship. *Journal of Religion, Disability, and Health, 15*(4), 431–436. https://doi.org/10.1080/15228967.2011.619341.

Renwick, R., DuBois, D., Cowen, J., Cameron, D., Schormans, A. F., & Rose, N. (2019). Voices of youths on engagement in community life: A theoretical framework of belonging. *Disability & Society, 34*(6), 945–971. https://doi.org/10.1080/09687599.2019.1583551.

Ryndak, D. L., Jackson, L., & Billingsley, F. (2000). Defining school inclusion for students with moderate to severe disabilities: What do the experts say? *Exceptionality, 8*(2), 101–116. https://doi.org/10.1207/S15327035EX0802_2.

Schalock, R. L., Brown, I., Brown, R., Cummins, R. A., Felce, D., Matikka, L., Keith, K. D., & Parmenter, T. (2002). Conceptualization, measurement, and application of quality of life for persons with intellectual disabilities: Report of an international panel of experts. *Mental Retardation, 40*(6), 457–470. https://doi.org/10.1352/0047-6765(2002)040<0457:CMAAOQ>2.0.CO;2.

Schnorr, R. F. (1990). "Peter? He comes and goes…": First graders' perspectives on a part-time mainstream student. *Journal of the Association for Persons with Severe Handicaps, 15*(4), 231–240. https://doi.org/10.1177/154079699001500402.

Schroeder, E. T., Carter, E. W., & Simplican, S. C. (2021). First-year orientation programs involving undergraduates with intellectual disability: Exploring barriers and belonging. *Journal of Postsecondary Education and Disability.*

Scior, K. (2011). Public awareness, attitudes and beliefs regarding intellectual disability: A systematic review. *Research in Developmental Disabilities, 32*(6), 2164–2182. https://doi.org/10.1016/j.ridd.2011.07.005.

Scior, K., & Werner, S. (2015). *Changing attitudes toward learning disabilities: A review of the evidence*. Mencap.

Simplican, S. C. (2019). Theorising community participation: Successful concept or empty buzzword? *Research and Practice in Intellectual and Developmental Disabilities, 6*(2), 116–124. https://doi.org/10.1080/23297018.2018.1503938.

Simplican, S. C., Leader, G., Kosciulek, J., & Leahy, M. (2015). Defining social inclusion of people with intellectual and developmental disabilities: An ecological model of social networks and community participation. *Research in Developmental Disabilities, 38*, 18–29. https://doi.org/10.1016/j.ridd.2014.10.008.

Siperstein, G. N., Norins, J., Corbin, S., & Shriver, T. (2003). *Multinational study of attitudes toward individuals with intellectual disabilities*. Special Olympics International.

Siperstein, G. N., Norins, J., & Mohler, A. (2007). Social acceptance and attitude change: Fifty years of research. In J. W. Jacobson, J. A. Mulick, & J. Rojahn (Eds.), *Handbook of intellectual and developmental disabilities* (pp. 133–154). Springer.

Smith, L., Wedgwood, N., Llewellyn, G., & Shuttleworth, R. (2015). Sport in the lives of young people with intellectual disabilities: Negotiating disability, identity and belonging. *Journal of Sport for Development, 3*(5), 61–70. https://jsfd.org/2015/12/05/sport-in-the-lives-of-young-people-with-intellectual-disabilities-negotiating-disability-identity-and-belonging/.

Strnadová, I., Johnson, K., & Walmsley, J. (2018). "... but if you're afraid of things, how are you meant to belong?" What belonging means to people with intellectual disabilities? *Journal of Applied Research in Intellectual Disabilities, 31*(6), 1091–1102. https://doi.org/10.1111/jar.12469.

Swinton, J. (2012). From inclusion to belonging: A practical theology of community, disability, and humanness. *Journal of Religion, Disability, & Health, 16*(2), 172–190. https://doi.org/10.1080/15228967.2012.676243.

Thompson, J. R., Schalock, R. L., Agosta, J., Teninty, L., & Fortune, J. (2014). How the supports paradigm is transforming the developmental disabilities service system. *Inclusion, 2*(2), 86–99. https://doi.org/10.1352/2326-6988-2.2.86.

Travers, H., & Carter, E. W. (2021). A systematic review of how peer-mediated interventions impact students without disabilities. *Remedial and Special Education*, Advance online publication. https://doi.org/10.1177/0741932521989414.

Tucker, E. C., Jones, J. L., Gallus, K. L., Emerson, S. R., & Manning-Ouellette, A. L. (2020). *Let's Take A Walk*: Exploring intellectual disability as diversity in higher education. *Journal of College and Character, 21*(3), 157–170. https://doi.org/10.1080/2194587X.2020.1781659.

U.S. Department of Education. (2017). *Child count and educational environments* [raw data]. https://www2.ed.gov/programs/osepidea/618-data/state-level-data-files/.

U.S. Department of Education. (2020). *The condition of education*. Author.

van Alphen, L. M., Dijker, A. J. M., Van Den Borne, H. H. W., & Curfs, L. M. G. (2009). The significance of neighbours: Views and experiences of people with intellectual disability on neighbouring. *Journal of Intellectual Disability Research, 53*(8), 745–757. https://doi.org/10.1111/j.1365-2788.2009.01188.x.

Vicente, E., Guillén, V. M., Gómez, L. E., Ibáñez, A., & Sánchez, S. (2018). What do stakeholders understand by self-determination? Consensus for its evaluation. *Journal of Applied Research in Intellectual Disabilities, 32*(1), 206–218. https://doi.org/10.1111/jar.12523.

Wehmeyer, M. L. (Ed.). (2013). The story of intellectual disability: An evolution of meaning, understanding, and public perception. Brookes.

Wehmeyer, M. L., Shogren, K. A., Little, T. D., & Lopez, S. J. (Eds.). (2017). *Development of self-determination through the life-course*. Springer.

Wentzel, K. R. (2017). Peer relationships, motivation, and academic performance at school. In A. J. Elliot, C. S. Dweck, & D. S. Yeager (Eds.), *Handbook of competence and motivation: Theory and application (pp. 586–603)*. Guilford Press.

Winsor, J., Timmons, J., Butterworth, J., Migliore, A., Domin, D., Zalewska, A., & Shepard, J. (2018). *StateData: The national report on employment services and outcomes*. University of Massachusetts Boston, Institute for Community Inclusion.

Wolfensberger, W. (1983). Social role valorization: A proposed new term for the principle of normalization. *Mental Retardation, 21*(6), 234–239. https://doi.org/10.1352/1934-9556-49.6.435.

Zuna, N., Summers, J. A., Turnbull, A. P., Hu, X., & Xu, S. (2010). Theorizing about family quality of life. In R. Kober (Ed.), *Enhancing the quality of life of people with intellectual disabilities* (pp. 241–278). Springer.

Chapter 3
Trusting Partnerships and Belonging for Families of Students with Disabilities

Ann Turnbull and Rud Turnbull

The roles of families of students with disabilities have significantly changed over the last 75 years as societal and cultural expectations evolved (Turnbull et al., 2015). Table 3.1 highlights eight key roles families have taken on as they navigate the educational system alongside their children. As parents of our son, Jay (1967–2009), who experienced intellectual and developmental disabilities, we assumed many of these roles. Within these roles, the major catalysts for rebalancing power between families and professionals occurred when The Arc of the USA (https://thearc.org/) was formed in the 1950s (role 3) and when the Individuals with Disabilities Education Act (IDEA) was passed in 1975 (roles 6 and 7). The eight roles can be subdivided into two major time frames: pre-IDEA (roles 1–6) and post-IDEA (roles 7–8). IDEA is the federal law that requires educational professionals to provide multidisciplinary services to infants and toddlers (birth through 2) with disabilities and a free appropriate public education to children and youth with disabilities, ages 3–21.

3.1 One Family's Story: How Family Roles Are Enacted

Our story is just a small history of family life before the Congress enacted IDEA. Jay was Rud's son from a previous marriage and was 6 when we married. At Jay's birth, physicians at a nationally top-ranked medical school advised Rud and Jay's

A. Turnbull (Retired) (✉) · R. Turnbull (Retired)
University of Kansas, Pittsboro, NC, USA
e-mail: turnbull@ku.edu

J. L. Jones, K. L. Gallus (eds.), *Belonging and Resilience in Individuals with Developmental Disabilities*, Emerging Issues in Family and Individual Resilience, https://doi.org/10.1007/978-3-030-81277-5_3

Table 3.1 Roles of families of students with disabilities

Family role	Description
1. Cause of their child's disability	Families were often blamed for causing their child's disability through bad parenting, especially related to autism
2. Recipients of professionals' decisions	Families were expected to adhere to the advice of professionals which often included institutionalizing their young child to "prevent the child from being a burden" to other family members
3. Organization members	Families banded together and founded The Arc of the USA (originally it had the now "outdated" name of the Association for Retarded Children) in the 1950s which over the years has advocated for equality of opportunity for individuals with intellectual and developmental disorders (IDD)
4. Service developers	Largely through organizational efforts, families developed programs to provide educational services to children with IDD who were excluded from public school
5. Teachers	Especially during preschool years, parents (typically mothers) were strongly encouraged to set aside daily time at home for teaching
6. Political advocates	Through leadership of The Arc of the USA in the late 1960s and early 1970s, parents brought state and federal lawsuits and advocated for state and federal legislation to mandate the rights of their children to attend public schools
7. Educational decision-makers	Through the passage of federal education legislation, now referred to as the Individuals with Disabilities Education Act (IDEA), students had the right to receive a free appropriate public education, and their parents had the right to share decision-making with educators in multiple ways, primarily through participating in the individualized education program (IEP) meeting
8. Trusted partners	The contemporary role for families is to enter into trusted partnerships with professionals in working together to ensure that students have an appropriately ambitious public education

Note. Adapted from Turnbull, A. P., Turnbull, H. R., Erwin, E., & Soodak, L., & Shogren, K. (2015). *Families, professionals, and exceptionality: Positive outcomes through partnerships and trust* (7th ed.). Pearson

biological mother that they should institutionalize Jay, essentially, stating that Jay did not belong with his family and his parents did not belong with him (role 2). They declined that advice; however, they ended up struggling with the lack of sufficient community resources.

3.1.1 Advocating for an Education

When Jay was 6 years old, we were back-to-back presidents of a local chapter of The Arc (role 3), spending many hours every week on organizational housekeeping (role 3), as well as advocacy for educational and adult services (roles 3 and 4). The public school system in the university community in which we lived did not provide any educational services for Jay or peers with similar educational needs. In fact, the school superintendent told us that if we would (a) obtain a grant to cover the salaries of a teacher and teacher aide, (b) recruit qualified educators for these two positions, and (c) identify six to eight other children with similar needs (role 4), he would direct the custodian to clear out the storage room in the administration building and set up a classroom in that space. He appeared to believe that this was a reasonable request of families of children with disabilities, failing to acknowledge the overt discrimination associated with his expectation of family rather than system responsibility. In fact, it was our impression that he presumed we should be grateful for the opportunity to provide the "free labor" to set up the class and for Jay to start school in an administration building that was filled with offices for adults and no other classrooms for children.

3.1.2 Advocating for Legislation

3.1.2.1 IDEA and the Individual Education Program

In the mid-1970s, Rud was the primary draftsman of the North Carolina special education law and lobbied relentlessly for its passage in the state legislature (role 6). We also worked with our congressional staff to attain their support for IDEA. Rud was on the team to draft federal regulations, especially in regard to the topic of procedural due process—the system of checks and balances when families and professionals disagree (role 6). During this time, we became keenly aware of the pervasive discrimination that we and other families whose children had IDD experienced. Our families had to work relentlessly for opportunities across all sectors of supports and services (e.g., school access, religious education, community recreation); whereas, our friends whose children did not have IDD took for granted that their children would have educational/community supports and services.

Passed originally in 1975, as the Education for All Handicapped Children Act (PL 94-142), IDEA mandates that students with disabilities receive a free appropriate public education. IDEA operationalizes the meaning of *appropriate* primarily through the development and implementation of the individualized education program (IEP). IDEA specifies that the IEP is a written document that outlines the annual educational program for students with disabilities including current levels of performance, annual goals, placement in the least restrictive settings, nature and frequency of services, and progress monitoring. The components of the IEP includes annual goals, benchmarks to reach the goals (required only for students with significant disabilities), nature of supplementary aids/services and related services, and placement determination in the least restrictive environmental setting. Additionally, IDEA sets forth the required participants for IEP development that include the student's parents, the student when appropriate, two teachers (one special educator and one general educator), an educator qualified to provide or supervise special education with knowledge about the general education curriculum and school resources, an individual who can interpret evaluation results, and other individuals with expertise invited by the parents or school personnel. Thus, the annual meeting to develop the IEP is the primary context for parents being educational decision-makers in seeking to ensure that their children receive an appropriate education (role 7).

3.1.2.2 Supreme Court Interpretation of IDEA

In 2017, the Supreme Court heard a case brought by the parents of Endrew, a boy with autism, who contended that his school failed to provide him with an appropriate education, as required by IDEA (Turnbull et al., 2017). Although Endrew's parents lost their claim at four lower hearings/reviews/courts, in the decision of *Endrew F. v. Douglas County School District RE-1* (2017), the Supreme Court issued a unanimous decision that students with disabilities are entitled to not only an appropriate education but rather an "ambitiously appropriate education." Thus, the Supreme Court strengthened the basis on which IEP teams comprised of families and professionals must make decisions that ensure progress for students with disabilities.

3.1.2.3 IDEA and Family-Professional Partnerships

The initial congressional expectation was that parents would be equal participants with professionals in making joint educational decisions within the IEP conference (Turnbull et al. 2007b) (role 7). However, a 16-year comprehensive review of research on IEP development concluded "the federal intention of parents and guardians being equal partners in collaborating with schools to develop IEPs is not being realized" (Blackwell & Rossetti, 2014, p. 11). Blackwell and Rossetti described common themes within IEPs of professionals dominating decision-making while parents were relegated to more passive roles. Across all disabilities, parents of color whose incomes fall below $25,000 are the least likely to attend IEP conferences (Wagner et al., 2012). Furthermore, compared to parents of students with other disabilities, parents of students with IDD are less likely to attend IEP conferences and report experiencing less satisfaction with their participation (Wagner et al., 2012).

Four decades after the passing of IDEA, parents of students with IDD repeatedly voice experiences of feeling like outsiders at their children's IEP meetings (see Wang et al., 2004). Common narratives about the power dynamics of IEP meetings highlight that many parents experience a sense of isolation rather than a sense of belonging. The most contemporary role for families (role 8) in need of full implementation is for families and professionals to experience trusting partnerships. The operationalization of this role through the Sunshine Model of Trusting Family-Professional Partnerships and its' alignment with the construct of belonging (Carter, 2016) are the focus of the remainder of this chapter.

3.2 Facilitating Resilience Through Trusted Family-Professional Partnerships: The Sunshine Model

We developed the Sunshine Model as a conceptual model to illustrate the centrality of trusted family-professional partnerships for meeting the needs of children with disabilities (see Fig. 3.1). Within the model, *partnership* refers to relationships in which individuals and/or entities enact joint rights and responsibilities in a cooperative manner, and *trust* refers to having confidence in someone's reliability, judgment, and word to act in the best interest of the person (Turnbull et al., 2022). Therefore, *trusting family-professional partnerships* in educational contexts are characterized by an alliance in which families and professionals confidently rely on each other's word, judgment, and wise actions to increase benefits for students and themselves.

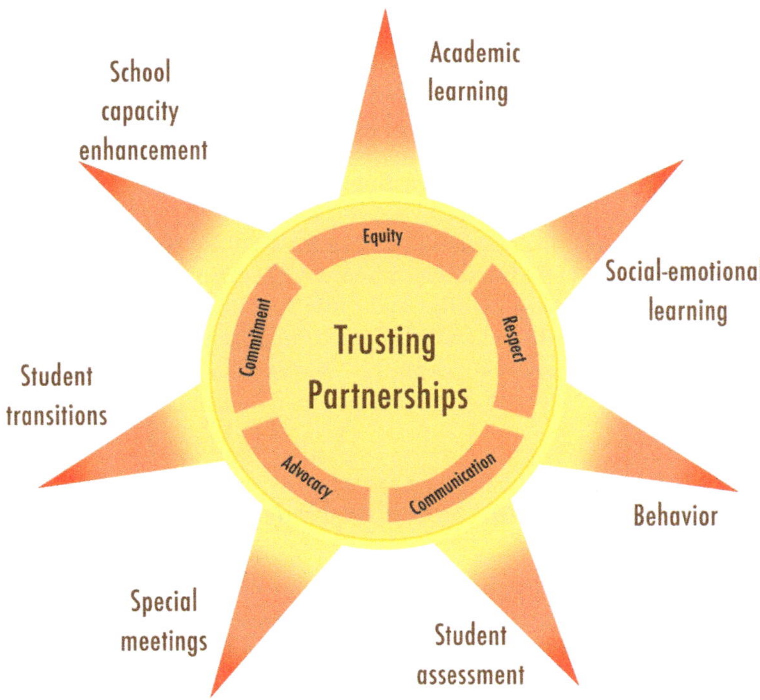

Fig. 3.1 Sunshine Model of Trusting Family-Professional Partnerships
Note. Reprinted with permission from Ann Turnbull. Originally published in: Turnbull, A. P., Turnbull, H. R., Francis, G., Burke, M., Kyzar, K. K., Haines, S., Gershwin, T., Shepard, K., Holdren, N., & Singer, G. (2022). *Families and professionals: Trusting partnerships in general and special education* (8th ed.). Pearson

3.2.1 Components of the Sunshine Model

The Sunshine Model conceptualizes five dimensions and seven opportunities for trusting partnerships. The five dimensions within the center of the sun (see Fig. 3.1) should be infused into each opportunity to foster trusting partnerships between and among families and professionals.

3.2.1.1 Five Dimensions of Trusting Partnerships

The core of the Sunshine Model is trust. Families and professionals can and should build trust with each other through the enactment of the five dimensions—equity, respect, communication, advocacy, and commitment. Table 3.2 includes definitions and indicators of each of the five dimensions (see bolded information in Table 3.2). These dimensions largely represent how families and professionals should interact with each other. Each dimension contributes to trust; yet it is only through enacting all five dimensions that trust can be actualized.

3.2.1.2 Seven Opportunities for Trusting Partnerships

As contrasted with the five dimensions focused on the foundations of trusting partnerships, the seven opportunities represent seven occasions for shared decision-making between and among families and professionals. The sunrays in Fig. 3.1 identify these opportunities as *academic learning*, *social-emotional learning*, *behavior*, *assessment*, *special meetings*, *transitions*, and *school capacity enhancement*.

3.2.2 Development of the Sunshine Model

Three strands of inquiry guided the development of the Sunshine Model. The first strand was comprised of a comprehensive qualitative inquiry and national survey resulting in the development of the Beach Center Family-Professional Partnership Scale, available free of charge for ongoing partnership research (https://beachcenter.lsi.ku.edu/beach-families/) (Blue-Banning et al., 2004; Summers et al. 2005a, b). The second strand of research focused on the effect of advocacy on families indicating the high level of stress that engaging in advocacy produces (Wang et al., 2004; Burke & Hodapp, 2014). The third research strand focused on the necessity for trust. Henderson and Mapp (2002) conducted a comprehensive review of 51 studies focusing on the impact of family/school/community connections on student achievement. They concluded that "building trusting collaborative relationships" (p. 7) was the key factor that enabled these connections to result in positive student outcomes.

Table 3.2 Definitions and indicators of the Sunshine Model's five dimensions of partnership

Partnership dimension	Definition, indicators, and examples
Equity	Moving beyond "equality" to apply intensive levels of support calibrated to needs, concerns, and resources that typically occur in light of systemic barriers
	Get to know families' preferences for communication—at parent-teacher conferences at the beginning of the school year, schedule extra time for parents who don't speak English, including Ms. Pérez; explore preferences for her communication from the outset rather than waiting until preparing for the IEP meeting
	Capitalize upon specialized resources—become familiar with community resources, especially those for families who face systemic barriers; ask Ms. Perez if prior to Alfredo's IEP meeting if she would like to meet with a Spanish-speaking parent from a parent advocacy program who could share her previous experiences in IEP meetings
	Make the least dangerous assumption about likely outcomes—examine and work to eliminate your own implicit biases; believe that Ms. Perez as a Spanish-speaking, single mother will be a valued partner in ensuring that Alfredo receives an ambitiously appropriate educational program and that Alfredo will meet high expectations
Respect	Conveying a sense of admiration for good or valuable qualities and also having genuine concern for families' needs and feelings
	Celebrate student and family strengths—make a habit of starting interactions with a focus on strengths; begin the IEP meeting by sharing with Ms. Perez positive things that Alfredo says at school about her and his family life, as well as highlighting Alfredo's strengths
	Be empathetic by relating to families' feelings and experiences—be sensitive to the emotional impact of the evaluation results and disability labels; relate to Ms. Perez' worry about Alfredo and the implications of his disabilities on his educational and adult success.
	Honor families' culture by reflecting on and addressing your own cultural lens—expand your own non-biased knowledge about diverse cultural circumstances and their educational impact; regarding Ms. Perez, expand your knowledge of the impact of immigration on family life and the pressures of working the night shift in a meat-packing plant
Communication	Engaging in culturally responsive and positive interactions that are reciprocal, frequent, and regular
	Listen through nonverbal and verbal listening behaviors—ask families open-ended questions and give undivided attention when they respond; invite Ms. Perez to share her concerns about Alfredo's education
	Connect through validating perspectives and emotions—affirm families' perspectives by expressing understanding and being nonjudgmental; address Ms. Perez' priority concerns, even if they differ from professional concerns
	Express by letting families know what to expect—share information with families in advance of the IEP meeting to enable them to lower anxiety and to be more confident; meet with Ms. Perez with an interpreter in advance of the IEP meeting to explain what will happen and to answer her questions; encourage her to consider inviting her aunt or anyone else to the meeting whose presence can result in an appropriately ambitious plan for Alfredo

(continued)

Table 3.2 (continued)

Partnership dimension	Definition, indicators, and examples
Advocacy	Taking action to solve problems or remove barriers in order to accomplish valued outcomes
	Develop viewpoints on key issues—recognize the systemic barriers many families face, including Ms. Perez, concerning the logistics that typically accompany families' roles in the education of their children and recognize the accountability of professionals as well as families in overcoming these
	Pinpoint and document concerns—for IEP conferences, develop a nonjudgmental understanding of systemic barriers to trusting partnerships; for Ms. Perez talk with her about her access to transportation and her time availability, given her sleep schedule during the day in light of her night working schedule
	Take action to find reasonable solutions—work with the principal and school social worker, as well as community resource agencies, to find transportation options for families to attend school meetings and activities; and work with Ms. Perez individually to ensure she can attend the meeting at school or hold the meeting at a community location for which public transportation is available; schedule the meeting at a time that is convenient for her
Commitment	Making deliberate choices to prioritize and value partnerships, as well as to assume responsibility for partnership outcomes
	Define goals and rationales for expanding your partnership commitment—recognize that developing trusting partnerships with families for the IEP process requires continuous reflection and learning; seek to "stand in Ms. Perez' shoes," as well as the "shoes" of other families, and determine what professional partnership approaches/skills would have the most favorable outcomes for them
	Develop and implement reasonable action plans to improve partnership outcomes—given one's own need for improvement with partnerships, locate and engage with opportunities and resources for professional development to expand competence and confidence; regarding Ms. Perez ensure competence and confidence in working with interpreters and being responsive to her need to sleep during times that many school activities are scheduled
	Evaluate outcomes and make improvements—seek feedback from families on partnership strategies and outcomes and act on their input; specifically ask Ms. Perez what partnership strategies she finds most and least helpful and whether or not she perceives that partnerships have been beneficial for her and Alfredo; respond to her feedback with responsive enhancements

Note. Adapted from: Turnbull, A. P., Turnbull, H. R., Francis, G., Burke, M., Kyzar, K. K., Haines, S., Gershwin, T., Shepard, K., Holdren, N., & Singer, G. (2022). *Families and professionals: Trusting partnerships in general and special education.* (8th ed.). Pearson

3.3 Fostering Belonging and Resilience Through Trusting Partnerships

Consider third grader, Alfredo, and his mother, Ms. Perez. Alfredo was recently evaluated for a disability based on academic and behavioral concerns. The psychological, educational, and behavioral assessments indicate that Alfredo has autism and intellectual disability. The next step in the IDEA process is a meeting between Ms. Perez and school personnel to review Alfredo's evaluation results and develop his IEP. Ms. Perez is a single mother who immigrated from Mexico without documentation, speaks Spanish as her primary language, and works in a meat-packing factory on the night shift. She lives with her aunt who cares for Alfredo when she is at work. Table 3.2 further illustrates how the five dimensions of partnership can be infused into an IEP meeting with Ms. Perez, transforming the IEP meeting from merely having Ms. Perez present at the meeting in a passive role to creating the opportunity for her to experience a trusted partnership where belonging and resilience can be actualized.

We conceptualize *belonging* as a necessary characteristic for children—and families—to experience resilience. Carter's (2016) explication of belonging with its ten dimensions has significantly contributed to our thinking in terms of enhancing the potential outcomes of the Sunshine Model. As we described earlier, students are the intended primary beneficiaries of trusted partnerships in schools. One of the seven partnership opportunities is social-emotional learning. As families and professionals work together to develop, implement, and monitor each student's social-emotional learning, it is a propitious time to focus directly on the current nature of students' belonging and how belonging can be enhanced. Additionally, there are ways to enhance students' belonging in each of the other six partnership opportunities: academic learning, behavior, assessment, special meetings, transitions, and school capacity enhancement. The Sunshine Model has the potential for fostering belonging in schools for families at the individual family level as well as at the collective school level.

3.3.1 *Individual Family Level in Schools*

The Sunshine Model's seven opportunities for partnerships provide multiple occasions and contexts for families "to be needed" (Carter's ninth dimension). Carter (2016) characterizes being needed as "…a real reciprocity, whereby each person both brings to and receives from the relationship" (p. 177). Let's return to the example of Ms. Perez and the way that professionals enact the five dimensions—equity, respect, communication, advocacy, and commitment—in order to actualize a trusting partnership with her in the context of the IEP meeting. She is "needed" in the development of Alfredo's IEP in order to ensure that the best possible decisions are made that will lead to the creation of his appropriately ambitious education. By enacting proactive partnership strategies, professionals and Ms. Perez transform her role from mere attendance (belonging dimension 1) to being needed (belonging dimension 9).

The Sunshine Model provides numerous additional opportunities for Ms. Perez "to be needed" beyond the IEP meeting. As the model is fully implemented, outcomes of the trusting partnership would include Ms. Perez being present, invited, welcomed, known, accepted, supported, cared for, and befriended (Carter, 2016). Thus, it is likely that she will experience belonging across nine of the ten dimensions.

3.3.2 Collective School Level

Consider the effect of a whole-school approach in which every family in the school—families of children with and without disabilities—and every professional experience the benefits of trusting partnerships. On several occasions, I (AT) had the privilege of visiting a school that has taken trusting partnerships to the collective school level. A charter school in Los Angeles, WISH, serves students from transitional K through grade 12. It is noteworthy that WISH is also a fully inclusive school. During these visits I conducted focus groups with parents of students with and without disabilities. The key word used in focus groups by families to describe the culture at WISH was "community." Parents offered various descriptors of community including a "warm atmosphere," "strong partnerships," "valuing diversity," "feeling safe," "everyone belonging," "everyone supported," "having no cliques," and "experiencing social justice." One parent described it as follows:

> This sense of community within the schools is just absolutely crucial…and that is something very unique at WISH. The families feel welcomed and have an opportunity any day, any time to make a suggestion on something. That there is a place for children of all abilities and all disabilities and that being in the same place to not only be able to be different but to be respected while you're being different.

With enthusiasm and excitement, parents described countless ways that they enjoyed enhancing school capacity and considered it their opportunity to "give back," for example, with a student focus (e.g., volunteering in classrooms to help with academic instruction, social development, and behavioral expectations); a teacher and teacher aide focus (e.g., grading papers, developing materials for art projects, designing bulletin boards); an administrator focus (e.g., fundraising, planning the new charter petition for the middle and high school); and a community focus (e.g., facilitating community projects such as environmental cleanup and 5K run).

Parents described that there is not just a willingness but indeed an eagerness to be as helpful as possible to teachers as a way of demonstrating reciprocity:

> Gosh, last year my kid's teacher sent an email out for "Oh we need this for birthdays of the month." And I swear that if it took more than 10 minutes to get back online, you were not

> gonna get on the list of stuff to contribute. Right, it's crazy. But as far as community goes, building that community, I honestly don't know what the secret formula is. And, I've never been to a school like this.

As with all things at WISH, the bottom line of trusting partnerships is how students are affected. Several parents particularly pointed out how much it means to their children that they, as parents, are school partners. A father commented:

> There's this really, real community that we feel, and I think when the parents are here, it sends a message to the kids about how much they are loved and how much they are cared for, and I think it helps them to develop that same sense of community with the other students.

In summary, we are confident that all ten dimensions of belonging—including love—for students, families, teachers, teacher aides, and administrators are experienced at WISH across all grade levels, literally on a minute-by-minute basis.

3.3.3 Applications in Settings Outside of Schools

We believe that the five dimensions of partnerships apply across multiple contexts associated with student and family belonging and resilience. While partnership opportunities (represented by sunrays in Fig. 3.1) would change in light of the context, the five dimensions of equity, respect, communication, commitment, and advocacy remain relevant to fostering trusting partnerships with professionals. Further, given that trusting partnerships require reciprocity, we are eager to explore the development of resources to prepare families and students to extend the same five partnership dimensions to professionals, as well as to each other. In what ways can families, as well as students, incorporate into their professional interactions equity, respect, communication, advocacy, and commitment to increase the likelihood of positive outcomes for all?

3.4 Epilogue

At the beginning of this article, we shared the challenges we experienced in getting the public schools to enable our son, Jay, to be *present* as a public school student, the mere first dimension of belonging. We want to end with a description of the partnership that we experienced with Jay's teacher, Mary Morningstar, during his last year of public school education when he was 21. Mary and Ann wrote individual perspectives on the trusting partnership we shared during the 1987–1988 school year. Here is a segment of Ann's perspective:

> Mary quickly earned our confidence in terms of the programming that she was doing, and we were totally together in our values for integration, productivity, and independence…She

> got Jay established as a manager of the football team. She also helped facilitate relationships between Jay and typical students (an opportunity he had never really had before) by helping him dress "cool," walk "cool," and generally fit into the school. It was an incredible relief for our family to not feel that we had to advocate during every spare minute to ensure Jay's happiness and progress. We knew that Mary was doing a great job, and we could relax and spend time in family recreation rather than in evening advocacy meetings. What a relief from previous years!...She treated us, as Jay's parents, and his sisters, Amy and Kate, with respect and dignity...The happy memories of Jay's last year at Walt Whitman High school will forever be part of the legacy that we hope to pass on through our professional world to other families and educators. (Turnbull & Morningstar, 1993, p. 1)

Consistent with Carter's (2016) emphasis on reciprocity, Mary also benefitted from our trusting partnership. A segment of her perspectives is as follows:

> Ann mentioned that Jay was the manager of the football team, but what she left out was that Rud and Kate enthusiastically attended just about every game, both home and away. They were there not only to cheer on the Whitman Vikings but also to support Jay, and through Jay, me and my program...Knowing that Ann and Rud were there to support my efforts was the most critical component of Jay's successful year. Their involvement provided me with the sustenance to continue my efforts and to continue to improve my program. School- and community-based programs require more than an 8-hour school day. It touches the lives of not only the student and teacher but also the family, school friends, neighbors, employers, store workers, bus drivers, and all who come in contact with the student and family. Establishing a trusting mutually beneficial family-professional partnership requires much effort and skill, but the outcomes of such a relationship far outweigh the efforts. (Turnbull & Morningstar, 1993, p. 2)

While earlier we discussed how the implementation of the Sunshine Model may lead to Ms. Perez experiencing nine of the Carter's ten dimensions of belonging, our story with Mary highlights the love that can emerge between families and professional when trusting partnerships are realized. Grote and Frieze (1994) define friendship-based love as "a comfortable, affectionate, trusting love..., based on a deep sense of friendship and involving companionship and the enjoyment of common activities, mutual interests, and shared laughter" (p. 275). We can affirm with deep honesty that we have loved Mary for the last 32 years, since we were fortunate enough to first experience our trusting partnership with her. Furthermore, Jay loved her until literally his dying day, even his dying hour; and he now loves her to infinity. We are confident that the feeling is mutual. We know beyond a shadow of a doubt that Mary loved Jay in life and continues to love him in death, and she loves us as well. Nothing can change the reciprocity of this tenth dimension. Thank you, Dr. Carter, for reminding us all that the ultimate dimension of belonging is love. Perhaps, it is also the ultimate outcome of trusting partnerships, as it was for Mary, Jay, and the two of us.

Questions for Thought and Discussion

1. What is your vision of how trusting family-professional partnerships could be expanded to trusting student-family-professional partnerships?
2. Reflect on the dimensions and indicators in Table 3.2, giving particular attention to the commitment dimension. What are three action steps you can begin

implementing in your scholarship and practice that prioritize and value trusting partnerships?
3. How would consistent implementation of the Sunshine Model enhance individual, family, and community resilience?

References

Blackwell, W. H., & Rossetti, Z. S. (2014). The development of individualized education programs: Where have we been and where should we go now? *SAGE Open*, 1–15. https://doi.org/10.1177/2158244014530411.

Blue-Banning, M., Summers, J. A., Frankland, H. C., Nelson, L. L., & Beegle, G. (2004). Dimensions of family and professional partnerships: Constructive guidelines for collaboration. *Exceptional Children, 70*, 167–184. https://doi.org/10.1177/001440290407000203.

Burke, M. M., & Hodapp, R. M. (2014). Relating stress of mothers of children with developmental disabilities to family-school partnerships. *Intellectual and Developmental Disabilities, 52*, 13–23. https://doi.org/10.1352/1934-9556-52.1.13.

Carter, E. W. (2016). A place of belonging: Research at the intersection of faith and disability. *Review and Expositor, 113*, 167–180. https://doi.org/10.1177/0034637316637861.

Grote, N. K., & Frieze, I. H. (1994). The measurement of friendship-based love in intimate relationships. *Personal Relationships, 1*, 275–300. https://doi.org/10.1111/j.1475-6811.1994.tb00066.x.

Henderson, A. T., & Mapp, K. L. (2002). *A new wave of evidence: The impact of school, family, and community connections to student achievement*. National Center for Family & Community Connections with Schools.

Summers, J. A., Hoffman, L., Marquis, J., Turnbull, A., & Poston, D. (2005a). Relationship between parent satisfaction regarding partnerships with professionals and age of child. *Topics in Early Childhood Special Education, 25*, 48–58. https://doi.org/10.1177/02711214050250010501.

Summers, J. A., Hoffman, L., Marquis, J., Turnbull, A., Poston, D., & Nelson, L. L. (2005b). Measuring the quality of family-professional partnerships in special education services. *Exceptional Children, 72*, 65–81. https://doi.org/10.1177/001440290507200104.

Turnbull, A. P., & Morningstar, M. E. (1993). In M. E. Snell (Ed.), *Instruction of students with severe disabilities* (4th ed., pp. 1–60). Macmillan.

Turnbull, H. R., Stowe, M. J., & Huerta, N. E. (2007b). *Free appropriate public education: The law and children with disabilities* (7th ed.). Love Publishing.

Turnbull, A., Turnbull, R., Erwin, E. J., Soodak, L. C., & Shogren, K. A. (2015). *Families, professionals, and exceptionality: Positive outcomes through partnerships and trust* (7th ed.). Pearson.

Turnbull, H. R., Turnbull, A. P., & Cooper, D. H. (2017). The Supreme Court, *Endrew*, and the appropriate education of students with disabilities. *Exceptional Children, 84*, 124–140. https://doi.org/10.1177/0014402917734150..

Turnbull, A. P., Turnbull, H. R., Francis, G., Burke, M., Kyzar, K. K., Haines, S., Gershwin, T., Shepard, K., Holdren, N., & Singer, G. (2022). *Families and professionals: Trusting partnerships in general and special education* (8th ed.). Pearson.

Wagner, M., Newman, L., Cameto, R., Javitz, H., & Valdes, K. (2012). A national picture of parent and youth participation in IEP and transition planning meetings. *Journal of Disability Policy Studies, 23*, 140–155. https://doi.org/10.1177/1044207311425384.

Wang, M., Mannan, H., Poston, D., Turnbull, A. P., & Summers, J. A. (2004). Parents' perceptions of advocacy activities and their impact on family quality of life. *Research and Practice for Persons with Severe Disabilities, 29*, 144–155. https://doi.org/10.2511/rpsd.29.2.144.

Chapter 4
Using the Universal Design for Learning Framework to Understand the Power of Belonging

Loui Lord Nelson

Where do students exist? Students exist in classrooms or in spaces that are acting as classrooms (e.g., a gathering of students with a teacher under the shade of a tree). We tend to associate students with a formal space (i.e., kindergarten through high school and postsecondary settings) and as individuals led by teachers, professors, instructors, or facilitators.

Where do learners exist? Learners exist wherever learning is taking place, but this might or might not be within a formal space. A learner is someone who becomes curious about a topic or a skill and continues to gain information. A learner uses reliable resources to increase knowledge. A learner seeks out others who have information to offer. A learner understands that knowledge and skill are acquired over time and with practice and that learning something significant takes planning. There are three crucial pieces to understanding the definition of a learner. First, being a learner is not dependent upon the space. Second, the role of a learner does not cease when the teacher is gone. Third, every person is a learner. For these reasons, universal design for learning (UDL), the topic of this chapter, uses the term learner versus student. Thus, this chapter will use the term learner.

This chapter introduces the framework of UDL through the lens of supporting learners with intellectual or developmental disabilities (IDD) by way of belonging and building resilience. Broadly speaking, UDL is a framework filled with information on the best strategies, supports, and techniques to meet the needs of all learners. The framework is grounded by the anticipated and expected differences in how individuals learn and experience learning across a variety of contexts. No two learners are the same; we already know this, but there are classrooms that are still designed that way. Instead of thinking about how to design a space that is

L. L. Nelson (✉)
The UDL Approach, Indianapolis, IN, USA
e-mail: lordnelson@raiseinc.com

J. L. Jones, K. L. Gallus (eds.), *Belonging and Resilience in Individuals with Developmental Disabilities*, Emerging Issues in Family and Individual Resilience, https://doi.org/10.1007/978-3-030-81277-5_4

cognitively, physically, and emotionally accessible to all learners, lessons are planned with the curriculum in mind. The majority of learners are taught the same way. Other learners are pulled aside or completely out of the general education classroom to receive other support. But what if educators switched their attention to designing for all learners? In what ways would all learners sense of belonging grow? And how might a sense of belonging build resilience? The following case study offers an example of this.

4.1 A Case Study

Dominique teaches at an arts-integrated school in Baltimore, Maryland, that is racially, linguistically, and socioeconomically diverse and is inclusive of learners with disabilities, including learners with IDD. Her eighth grade classroom includes 35 learners including learners with IDD, English language learners, learners who have just moved to the United States, and learners who are gifted and talented. These descriptors are not exclusive to individual learners, either. For example, one learner does not use English as his primary language, and he is gifted in math.

Because it is an arts-integrated school, learners have always had art-related ways to explore, learn about, and demonstrate their connection to the topic or subject. The school also focuses on establishing a culture of curiosity, reflection, kindness, and persistence through restorative justice and practices that align with social-emotional skill-building. When we read, it is believed that our eyes and brain see combinations of letters and our brains recognize patterns that we know as words. This is the act of decoding. The act of comprehension is when we understand what that pattern of letters or words mean. When students have challenges in decoding, it can hamper their ability to comprehend, but when they are assisted with decoding, they have a better opportunity to comprehend.

Dominique noticed that she was not able to fully engage her learners in her English language arts classes. For example, her English language learners, some of her learners with disabilities, and other general education learners were overwhelmed when decoding, understanding the nuances of the English language, or digging into and discussing concepts such as narrative and plot. Other learners had different levels of understanding of grammar and writing. Keeping up with each of their needs was like trying to plug little holes in a large dam. While she was paying attention to the needs of one learner, seven other learners had seven other needs.

Dominique was introduced to universal design for learning and took hold of it. She was fascinated by the brain science behind it and joyfully recognized some of her teaching strategies and practices represented in the UDL graphic organizer. Beyond that, though, Dominique saw that UDL could help her develop lessons and an environment that would provide support for all of her learners upfront instead of the constant retrofitting she was doing. She could stop plugging up holes and instead fix the entire dam.

She decided to focus on the design of her upcoming poetry unit. She already knew her learners would create visual representations, but she also began thinking through what each of her learners would bring to the unit and the barriers her learners would experience during the unit. She wanted her learners to create a portfolio of poetry and art that told their stories. According to the state's educational standards, they needed to be able to express themselves through writing and performance, but she also knew she wanted them to gain a stronger sense of voice as well as a stronger sense of community in the classroom and the school.

The barriers Dominique identified across the entire class were a lack of grammatical and decoding skills to support the analyses of rigorous poems and the authorship skills necessary to create their own poems. She also identified a lack of organizational skills and long-term planning to create a portfolio of work and a general disinterest in poetry. Another barrier some of her learners faced was completing work quickly and efficiently, so they became bored and restless, leaving them disengaged in their learning environment. Finally, she knew many would comprehend the examples differently. For example, some of her learners with IDD might be more literal in their translation of poems as might some of her English learners, so she identified that as a need to be met.

Dominique was familiar with the accommodations (i.e., additional supports provided to students based on identified needs) within her learners' IEPs and found many of those were in line with the barriers other learners were experiencing. One of her learners named Barret utilized a communication system and an electric wheelchair, had limited use of his arms, and demonstrated lower cognitive skills than his peers on standardized assessments. Dominique knew he could participate in the unit, though. Sure, the accommodations Barret needed were in place, but many of his other accommodations were already blended into the environment, so Dominique knew he could be successful. For example, Barret needed more time to physically create or author products. In other environments, this need was turned into a barrier by teachers who put in place strict timelines and processes. In Dominique's classroom, though, Barret and some of his other classmates had the freedom to determine how best to use their time, so they could complete their project within the allotted amount of overall time. Dominique provided guidance in how to schedule their tasks and create checklists, so they could move through their tasks effectively. These were just some examples of how she was beginning to understand how our brains learn and how she could and should remove barriers to learning for all learners. Another way she lowered barriers was through choice.

First, Dominique added in choice where she could to increase autonomy and engagement. After setting guidelines and class-wide expectations, she let all learners assess and sit where they would work and learn best. Some learners struggled with this level of choice, so she was prepared with guidance for them. She also gave her learners a wide selection of poetry from which to choose and helped them choose what related to them both in experience and comprehension. The help she provided was styled after facilitation rather than a directive. For example, though she made suggestions, each learner made the final choice. To help them make that choice, she provided them with 15 different types of poetry forums and structures.

She also did a lot of modeling. For example, she modeled the analysis of multimedia poems, visual poems, rap, hip hop music, popular radio hits, TED talks, novels in verse, poetry via video, and spoken word. She broke the analysis process down into written and vocally recorded steps, so learners could reference them repeatedly in whatever way met their need.

Some of the learners were very interested in science, so she made sure they had materials to help them investigate what happens to the brain when you read poetry. To support their writing, she offered a variety of organizers digitally and on paper. She did explicit modeling of how to use the thesaurus, the dictionary, and translation tools on the Internet. Over time, she built layers that immersed all learners in the world of poetry and promoted optimal engagement. But she also made poetry accessible to all of her learners by ensuring they had different ways to read (e.g., via decoding and via listening), write (e.g., via utensils, the keyboard, or speaking), and otherwise communicate their poetry (e.g., the use of the art options). Her goal was to make every learner feel a connection to poetry and feel capable of analyzing and authoring it. She provided clear and guiding feedback on their projects and writing along the way, encouraging them to improve their products over time. In each case, these supports and tools were made available to Barret. The paraprofessional assigned to Barret helped foster relationships between Barret and his peers by making sure that he was included in discussions, that he was utilizing the online and digital tools, and that he was meeting with his writing partner to assess both of their accomplishments for each person (all of the learners had writing partners).

When it came to expressing their poetry, they had multiple modalities from which to choose including PowerPoint, posters, and other visual arts (e.g., clay form, painting, drawing, and digital graphics). Barret decided to use PowerPoint and a digital paint application on the iPad to show his ideas. Every single learner presented their portfolio of poems to the class. They did this by displaying their visuals next to them and reading their poetry. English learners shared their work in their first language and in English. Barret worked with Dominique, the paraprofessional, and his parents to enter his poetry into the device and used a digital graphic program to project his art. Dominique taped her slide advancer to Barret's chair so he could forward the slides on his own command. Every learner told their own story through their poetry which raised the level of appreciation, understanding, and community throughout the classroom. Throughout this entire unit, every learner knew they belonged in that learning environment. Every learner was expected to be there and every learner was expected to participate. Every learner was expected to produce and every learner was supported to achieve. By designing for the learner variability that was present, Dominique established a clear sense of belonging and provided an environment that promoted resilience in learning, relationship building, and academic success.

This case study illustrates one teacher's implementation of a UDL in one particular context. Next, UDL is introduced through the findings of science and application. The remaining section shares how designing for belonging and resilience through UDL can benefit all learners, including those with IDD.

4.2 Universal Design for Learning

The universal design for learning is a multifaceted framework. Table 4.1 provides four descriptions to demonstrate the breadth of the framework. Each description notes that UDL supports all learners; there are no exceptions. All learners benefit from these collected practices because the practices were selected according to the way the brain is organized to learn (Rose & Strangman, 2007). From there, each description articulates certain dimensions.

The first description of UDL clarifies the use of evidence-based practices and innovations. The second description draws our attention to lowering barriers. The third reminds us that UDL should be utilized across all facets of education. The fourth is the densest, including the concepts of flexibility and high expectations, and articulates certain learner groups to ensure the understanding of the phrase "all learners." Ultimately, the proposed outcome for learners who experience lessons and learning environments designed using UDL is to gain skills associated with the traits of an expert learner. These traits include (a) identifying, understanding, and connecting with the purpose of learning; (b) understanding utilizing intrinsic and extrinsic motivation to achieve; (c) identifying resources to support learning; (d) understanding what tools and resources are needed to gain knowledge; (e) the ability to create a useful strategy; and (f) the ability create a goal and maintain the necessary focus to achieve that goal (CAST, 2018).

The image most often associated with UDL is the graphic organizer referred to as The Guidelines (CAST, 2018) (Fig. 4.1).

Table 4.1 Descriptions of the universal design for learning framework

Description 1	UDL is a collection of evidence-based practices and innovations that are organized according to anatomic and psychological brain functions which are part of how the brain learns (Meyer et al., 2014; Rose & Strangman, 2007). The intention is to provide educators guidance as they design their lessons and learning environments for all learners
Description 2	UDL shifts educators from not considering barriers when lesson planning to designing lessons and environments that are barrier-free, instructionally rich, and accessible (Nelson, 2021)
Description 3	UDL "involves planning and delivering programs with the needs of all learners in mind. It applies to all facets of education: from curriculum, assessment, and pedagogy to classroom and school design" (Mitchell, 2014, p. 236)
Description 4	According to the Higher Education Act of 2008 (20 U.S.C. 1003), the term "universal design for learning" means a scientifically valid framework for guiding educational practice that:
	(A) Provides flexibility in the way information is presented, in the ways learners respond or demonstrate knowledge and skills, and in the ways learners are engaged
	(B) Reduces barriers in instruction, provides appropriate accommodations, supports, and challenges and maintains high achievement expectations for all learners, including learners with disabilities and learners who are limited English proficient

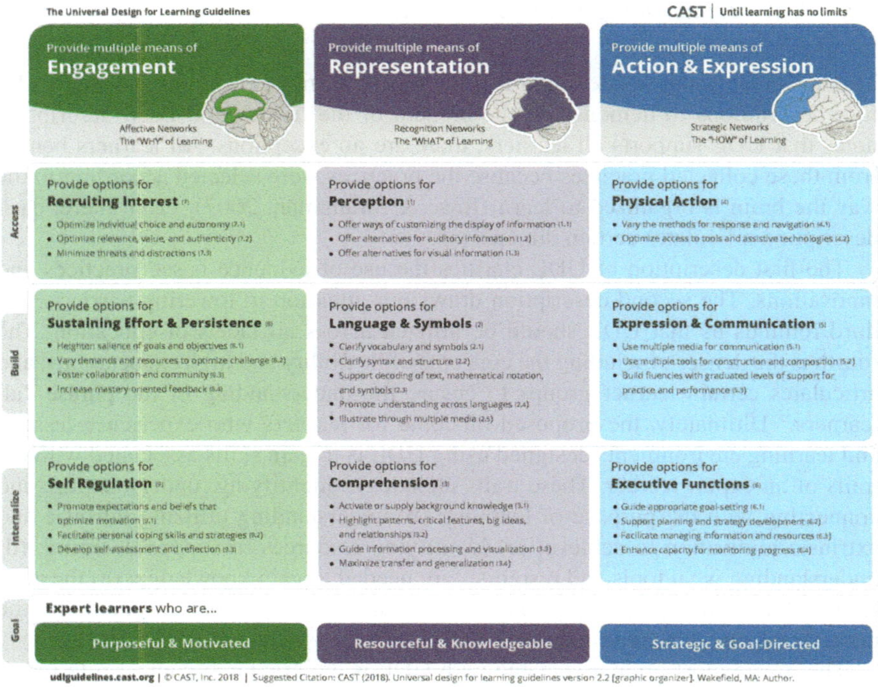
The Universal Design for Learning Guidelines
CAST | Until learning has no limits
Provide multiple means of
Engagement
Affective Networks
The "WHY" of Learning
Provide multiple means of
Representation
Recognition Networks
The "WHAT" of Learning
Provide multiple means of
Action & Expression
Strategic Networks
The "HOW" of Learning
Access
Provide options for
Recruiting Interest (7)
Optimize individual choice and autonomy (7.1)
Optimize relevance, value, and authenticity (7.2)
Minimize threats and distractions (7.3)
Provide options for
Perception (1)
Offer ways of customizing the display of information (1.1)
Offer alternatives for auditory information (1.2)
Offer alternatives for visual information (1.3)
Provide options for
Physical Action (4)
Vary the methods for response and navigation (4.1)
Optimize access to tools and assistive technologies (4.2)
Build
Provide options for
Sustaining Effort & Persistence (8)
Heighten salience of goals and objectives (8.1)
Vary demands and resources to optimize challenge (8.2)
Foster collaboration and community (8.3)
Increase mastery-oriented feedback (8.4)
Provide options for
Language & Symbols (2)
Clarify vocabulary and symbols (2.1)
Clarify syntax and structure (2.2)
Support decoding of text, mathematical notation, and symbols (2.3)
Promote understanding across languages (2.4)
Illustrate through multiple media (2.5)
Provide options for
Expression & Communication (5)
Use multiple media for communication (5.1)
Use multiple tools for construction and composition (5.2)
Build fluencies with graduated levels of support for practice and performance (5.3)
Internalize
Provide options for
Self Regulation (9)
Promote expectations and beliefs that optimize motivation (9.1)
Facilitate personal coping skills and strategies (9.2)
Develop self-assessment and reflection (9.3)
Provide options for
Comprehension (3)
Activate or supply background knowledge (3.1)
Highlight patterns, critical features, big ideas, and relationships (3.2)
Guide information processing and visualization (3.3)
Maximize transfer and generalization (3.4)
Provide options for
Executive Functions (6)
Guide appropriate goal-setting (6.1)
Support planning and strategy development (6.2)
Facilitate managing information and resources (6.3)
Enhance capacity for monitoring progress (6.4)
Goal
Expert learners who are...
Purposeful & Motivated
Resourceful & Knowledgeable
Strategic & Goal-Directed
udlguidelines.cast.org | © CAST, Inc. 2018 | Suggested Citation: CAST (2018). Universal design for learning guidelines version 2.2 [graphic organizer]. Wakefield, MA: Author.

Fig. 4.1 CAST's UDL guidelines. (© 2021 CAST. Used with permission. All rights reserved)

The three principles of engagement, representation, and action and expression provide an overall organization. In each of those columns are three guidelines (nine in total). Each guideline is further described by checkpoints. Some guidelines have three checkpoints, while others have five. There are 31 checkpoints in total. Each checkpoint, guideline, and principle are thoroughly defined using research from the fields of education, special education, psychology, cognitive psychology, and neuropsychology (Nelson, 2021). Educators use The Guidelines as a reference to design their learning environment and lessons, but it doesn't tell them everything there is to know about UDL nor does it prescribe how to design lessons or learning environments.

Educators not only use the UDL framework to design their lessons; they also use The Guidelines to design their learning environment. To do this successfully, it is important to understand the concept of learning environment and what a learning environment includes.

4.2.1 The Learning Environment

Typically, when we think of a place where learning takes place, we think of the classroom. From there, we think of books, pencils, pens, and digital tools (e.g., computers, tablets, apps, projectors, white boards). We think of desks, bookshelves, rugs, lamps, and cabinets. There are, however, other dynamics that expand the idea of a classroom to the concept of a learning environment.

First, the term *learning environment* broadens our thinking to go beyond the four walls of the classroom and recognize that learning can take place anywhere (Meyer et al., 2014; Nelson, 2021). Learning takes place in hallways, the office, conference rooms, the counselors' office, the bus, and in the community. Instead of limiting learning to a defined geographical space, we can expand our responsibility for and thinking about quality design.

Second, how we use the physical objects within the learning environment directly impacts the learners. Do the learners have access to learning materials when they need them? Do they have to request permission, or are there some resources that are always available? Do learners decide which resources they need to use or are they assigned resources? All of these questions return to the underlying concept of choice discussed above (Nelson, 2019).

Third, an often-forgotten but crucial component of any learning environment is the relationship learners have with one another and with the teacher. The interpersonal relationships teachers have with their learners is a critical factor in learner success (Hamre & Pianta, 2001; Whitted, 2011). How we design the learning environment directly impacts how learners learn because the environment is dynamic and the learner is dynamic (Meyer et al., 2014). To understand how the learner is dynamic, we need to return to the foundation of UDL: the brain.

4.2.2 The Learning Brain

In 1962, the Russian psychologist Vygotsky shared that learning is dependent upon our ability to engage with the learning task, recognize the information to be learned, and apply strategies to process that information (Rose & Strangman, 2007). He also understood that learning is social. While learning requires effort, barriers that prevent that development can be mitigated by working with others (e.g., other learners as well as educators) who are advanced in that task or skill (Levykh, 2008). His work was organized into three prerequisites for learning: engagement with the learning task; recognition of the information to be learned; and the application of strategies to process that information (Rose & Meyer, 2002). Using those prerequisites as a base, CAST grouped the characteristics and outcomes of the learning brain into three areas: the affective (engaging), recognition (recognizing), and strategic (identifying and using strategies) (Rose & Meyer, 2002; Rose & Strangman, 2007).

The affective networks, which align with the principle of engagement, are where we decide what matters to us and what actions to take (Damasio, 1994; Lane & Nadel, 2000; Ledoux, 2003; Panksepp, 1998; Rose & Dalton, 2007). These networks influence our everyday decision-making and actions due to emotional, motivation, and biological drivers (Immordino-Yang & Gotlieb, 2017). Examples of biological drivers include thirst or hunger. Our affective networks are also the door to our learning. When we are connected to and feel safe within an environment, learning is more accessible (Meyer et al., 2014). Threats can be external such as a loud environment where the learner cannot concentrate, or threats can be internalized. One example of an internalized threat is called stereotype threat. Stereotype threat occurs when individuals view themselves as part of a group and believe that failure might confirm negative stereotypes of that group and by extension, themselves (Hammer et al., 2016; Steele & Aronson, 1995). This belief keeps them from performing to their potential.

Seminal research conducted by Steele and Aronson (1995) showed that African-American learners experienced stereotype threat in their day-to-day coursework leads to an achievement gap. The research discovered that these learners saw their failure as a confirmation of the stereotype associated with all African-Americans. By providing the learners with several opportunities to write affirming statements of how they value something about themselves (e.g., a skill, a relationship they had with others, or another value), that achievement gap closed by over 40% (Cohen et al., 2006; Meyer et al., 2014). This demonstrates how the potency of our affective networks is tied to perception (e.g., learners' perception of task difficulty and its alignment with their culturally constructed identity) (Immordino-Yang & Gotlieb, 2017; Nasir, 2012). Our learning is impacted by how we perceive ourselves as learners.

Our recognition networks, which align with the principle of representation, guide us toward an understanding of our environment through the use of our senses, but they also work on prediction. These networks identify and predict straightforward and complex patterns like color, sound, smell, faces, words, letters, and even the difference between how two authors write (Meyer et al., 2014). In general, humans are often startled, though, when experiencing a cognitive awakening, leading to seeing something not seen first. For example, there is a famous image of a woman sitting at her dressing table and looking in a mirror. There is an alternate image within that picture. When we see it, we experience that jolt of recognition (Morales & Macpherson, 2017). Our learning is impacted by whether or not our recognition networks are provided substantial opportunities to tap into our patterns of prediction.

Our strategic networks, which align with the principle of action and expression, guide our goal-setting, planning, and execution, both mental and physical (Meyer et al., 2014). We act strategically. For example, why do we brush our teeth? We brush them to prevent tooth decay. For it to be its most effective, it is something we are supposed to do after each meal. The act of preventing tooth decay takes goal-setting (you brush your teeth after each meal), planning (you replace your toothbrush every 6 months, you purchase tooth paste when needed, and you set aside time after every meal to brush your teeth), and execution (you uncap the tooth paste tube, put the tooth paste on the brush, cap the tooth paste tube, brush your teeth, rinse your mouth, and rinse your toothbrush). Finally, you go to the dentist every 6 months, and you are told whether your brushing is effective. The focus here is on the strategy part of the task. This example includes all of the networks but focuses on the strategic parts. Our ability to grow our strategic networks impacts our ability to complete tasks successfully.

These networks are articulated as three different areas in the UDL framework for the purpose of definition and understanding. Our brain functions in both specialized ways and heterarchical, meaning there are specific areas where functions take place, but our brains are constantly predicting and anticipating what we will experience or do next (Meyer et al., 2014). This can occur from the top-down (i.e., brain to body) or from bottom-up, which is why it is heterarchical.

Understanding how the brain learns empowers educators to establish learning environments that support all three learning networks. Doing so allows learners, including those with IDD, have the opportunity to be included. By doing so, educators create the context for belonging and resilience.

4.3 Design for Learners with Intellectual and Developmental Disabilities: A Context for Belonging and Resilience

When the inclusion of learners with intellectual or developmental disabilities focuses solely on location, the burden for learning is placed on the learner – they must prove they can be successful utilizing the curriculum offered in that location (Jorgensen et al., 2007). In a location-focused model, the curriculum stays the same, and the learner is expected to either make the accommodations or leave that curriculum setting. This is a "one-size-fits-all" approach (Rose & Strangman, 2007). The UDL shifts this thinking. It commands that the curriculum meet the academic and social-emotional needs of all learners (Meyer et al., 2014). This is done by recognizing the barriers (i.e., the cognitive, physical, or emotional structures that prevent individuals from learning) present within the current environment and curriculum and weaving in options based on the UDL guidelines, so all learners can achieve the determined goal and gain skills toward becoming expert learners. The curriculum is now flexible and responds to each learner because it recognizes the uniqueness of each learner as that learner moves from one context to another (Meyer et al., 2014). Inherent within this shift is a shift toward belonging.

When the location and curriculum are locked together, learners are left out and are told implicitly and explicitly they do not belong in that location. When the focus shifts to the design of the curriculum, the uniqueness of each learner becomes an asset to the location. Every learner belongs. In addition, because every learner is enveloped within an environment designed using the UDL framework, they are provided learning opportunities and experiences that help them gain skills toward becoming expert learners. This means they are gaining resilience.

Educational resilience is defined as "the heightened likelihood of educational success despite personal vulnerabilities and adversities brought about by environmental conditions and experiences" (Wang et al., 1998, p. 2). Educators who implement the UDL recognize that the adversarial environmental conditions are the barriers. As exemplified within the case story that opened this chapter, though, lowering barriers did not equate to lowering rigor.

By implementing the UDL, Dominique removed barriers to learning for all of her learners and responded to their uniqueness by (a) designing the unit based on known and anticipated learner needs and (b) using flexible sources (e.g., a variety of tools, including digital resources) to create an environment that kept all of her learners connected to the learning and connected to one another. She was responding to the variability across learners by lowering barriers. As is true in all settings, when the rigor remains high and the barriers are lowered, learners are provided with experiences and challenges that leave them with feelings of accomplishment and resilience (Blackburn, 2013). This chapter continues by explaining the concepts of variability and barriers as they relate to UDL.

4.3.1 Variability and Barriers

4.3.1.1 Embracing Variability Through Universal Design for Learning

UDL stems from the premise that all of us learn differently based on the context (Meyer et al., 2014). We are accustomed to hearing that we are all different and we all learn differently, but the concept of variability takes it a step further. We each learn differently based on where we are, what we are learning, how we are feeling, and who is involved. Those four areas together are called context. Context is the influence an environment can have on a person and the process (Bronfenbrenner & Morris, 1998; Peets, 2009). In a video specifically addressing variability, Rose (2011) reminds us that the design of a lesson and the environment (the context) directly impacts how the learner gains access to and participates in learning so much so that "[l]earners of all ages, of all nationalities, of all types are highly variable. Whether they're disabled or not depends on their interaction with the context." This directly aligns with the social-ecological perspective of disability that there is a "complex interplay between a person and their environment" (Shogren, 2013, p. 3). In the case of variability, *interaction* or *interplay* determines whether or not a learner has access to participate, understand, and demonstrate growth in knowledge or experience. Disability is not removed; rather, the needs related to the disability are accommodated through the broad design of the lesson and learning environment. This creates an environment already primed to support accommodations that might be unique to the individual, such as the use of a particular type of chair, the use of headphones at all times, or a communication device. Communication devices are assistive technology that supports learners in communicating with others. No-tech options include an alphabet board a student uses to point to letters to spell out words.

High-tech options include computerized version of the alphabet board along and incorporate lists of words. Some devices are connected to switches so individuals who have limited use of their hands or feet can tap their head or chin against a pad or puff on a straw. In these cases, the pad or straw act as the mouse, and the individual can make the necessary choices. A communication system only replaces vocalized words. The individual is still in control of what they say and to whom they speak.

4.3.1.2 Removal of Barriers Through Universal Design for Learning

Returning to Dominique's design, she recognized the barriers her learners would likely experience and added in supports to help them move past those barriers. Rather than focusing on specific activities for individual learners, she designed the overall unit to accommodate the broad needs. Equally important, though, she designed the lesson and learning environment so the learners gained skills in choice-making and decision-making. Both skills sets are critically important to growth in self-determination (Agran et al., 2006; Shogren et al., 2004). In addition, many supports traditionally reserved for learners with intellectual and developmental disabilities (e.g., audio of text, print size, dictation, spaces with minimal disruptions, pacing structures, written instructions) were available to all learners with the purpose of helping each learner identify the supports they needed depending on the context. She planned for the known variability of her learners.

In other situations, learners who are excellent at decoding via reading with their eyes might choose to listen to poems because they discover they can hear the rhythm of the poem better. Without the ability to listen, their learning is minimized. In many cases, though, the assumption is made that a learner with strong decoding skills will be able to decipher a poem more easily than their peers who cannot decode well. As is true with all learners, their interaction with the context determines their level of learning. There are profound changes occurring in education based on our digitally networked and multimodal world so much so that the concepts of accessibility and accommodations are being redefined (Gregg, 2012; Meyer et al., 2014). These changes can equate to minimizing barriers for more learners. Next, this chapter investigates the interconnection of UDL, learners with IDD, belonging, and resilience.

4.3.2 Universal Design for Learning, Learners with Intellectual and Developmental Disabilities, Belonging, and Resilience

4.3.2.1 Research on Universal Design Learning and Learners with Intellectual and Developmental Disabilities

Researchers have examined the implementation of the UDL framework inclusive of learners with IDD (e.g., Browder et al., 2008; Coyne et al., 2017; Dymond et al., 2006; Lieber et al., 2008; Lowrey et al., 2017). Though the studies have varied in method, the number of participants, and purpose, the outcomes experienced by the learners with IDD were positive.

The design of a study done by Lowrey et al. (2017), though, allowed for a closer look at belonging. The researchers interviewed general education teachers in the United States and Canada experienced with the UDL framework and who taught in inclusive classrooms that included learners with intellectual disabilities. They examined the language used by the educators as representations of their underlying beliefs (Johnston, 2004) and found examples of language that supported and prohibited belonging. The language that supported belonging aligned with several of the checkpoints and guidelines under the UDL principle of engagement.

When referencing learners with IDD, teachers used language that emphasized learner comfort in asking others for help, learner-to-learner trust during station work, and the assignment of jobs during academic tasks (e.g., science experiments). Alternatively, these same teachers used language that prevented belonging. Phrases like "placing learners in your class" and "putting those learners in your room" reflected one teacher's view that the learners were not true members of that learning community (p. 18). Another teacher used age as a descriptor of ability: "I have a set of twins that are in grade eight but mentally they are about three years old" (p. 18). Finally, the types of jobs that were assigned to learners with IDD were basic and not meaningful, including jobs that kept them busy while the other learners completed academic tasks (e.g., filling in graphs). While the general educators involved in this study identified ways to promote belonging in association with the UDL framework, and more specifically the principle of engagement, their language did not communicate a full understanding of how to support the belonging of learners with IDD.

This disconnect is further articulated in a study conducted with Australian teachers (Capp, 2017). The researcher created a tool to measure the confidence expressed by teachers in their implementation of the UDL framework. Capp converted the principles, guidelines, and checkpoints into a questionnaire designed using a five-point Likert scale: "(1) very unconfident, (2) not confident, (3) unsure, (4) confident, and (5) very confident" (p. 5). The results showed that teachers in both primary grades (grade four to grade six) and secondary (grades seven to twelve) felt the least confident about the checkpoints under engagement. Overall, teachers were more comfortable with implementing the principle of representation than they were with the principles of action and expression or the principle of engagement. They were the least comfortable implementing the checkpoints under the principle of engagement. Though this is only one study and it was not specific to the inclusion of learners with IDD, the implications of this study on supporting learners with disabilities to have a sense of belonging are significant.

As stated earlier, our emotional centers (which are aligned with the principle of engagement) are the gateway to learning as well as the most directly related to the emotion of belonging. When teachers do not understand the importance of, the reason for, and/or the purpose of the principle of engagement, all learners are affected, but learners with IDD are affected even more. The potential for emotional disconnect and a sense of not belonging is genuine. In addition, resilience, which is closely linked to the principle of engagement, is not fostered. Instead, educators can use the principle of engagement to foster resilience. Two guidelines within that principle have clear connections to resilience and can be applied: sustaining effort and persistence and self-regulation. Table 4.2 articulates how specific checkpoints within these two guidelines guide educators to provide opportunities to build resilience.

4.3.2.2 The Learning Environment: Affective Networks, Engagement, and Belonging

Carter's (2016) work investigates the intersection of faith and disability and examines the act of belonging. In Chapter 1 of this collection, Carter takes the ten dimensions of belonging, articulating how each intersects and builds on the other until the individual reaches the point of feeling loved. These ten dimensions also inform the discussion of community in the educational setting. For example, the current

Table 4.2 Connecting two universal design for learning guidelines to resilience

Guideline	Checkpoint	Opportunities to build resilience
Sustaining effort and persistence	Varied demands and resources to optimize challenge	The barriers are lowered via the options provided, but rigor is maintained. Learners learn to choose the resources that will help them meet their goals
	Foster collaboration and community	Learners receive guidance on how to utilize partnerships with others to gain the information, skills, and knowledge they need. Learners gain communication and connection skills
	Increase mastery-oriented feedback	Learners receive specific and detailed feedback designed to direct them toward improved performance and outcomes. Students learn to accept and utilize this feedback
Self-regulation	Promote expectations and beliefs that optimize motivation	Learners are placed in a motivating environment but also learn skills and tools that help them learn how to self-motivate
	Facilitate personal coping skills and strategies	Learners are guided in their use and adoption of coping skills and strategies. They are encouraged to use these skills within and outside of academic settings
	Develop self-assessment and reflection	Learners are provided tools that guide self-assessment and reflection and are provided prompts and suggestions on how to use those tools both inside and outside of academic settings

conversations about inclusion in churches (i.e., the concept of place is stronger than the concept of belonging) mirror the historical conversations held about inclusion in K-12 schools. Early efforts in education focused on the physical placement of learners (Artiles, 2011), but there has been a shift. With its focus on flexible tools, strategies, and pathways to mastering learning goals, UDL supports this shift because it "has the potential to expand options for learners with ID in general education settings" (Rao et al., 2017, p. 37) which provides a pathway toward meaningful participation for all learners. This includes their engagement which is guided by the affective networks.

The work of neuropsychologists is to establish a deeper understanding of the connection between our neuronal experiences (the activity in our brains) and our emotional experiences (Immordino-Yang & Gotlieb, 2017; Immordino-Yang & Damasio, 2011). Those who are interested in the connection to education use a cross-examination of methods including neuroimaging, psychophysiological recording (e.g., change of body temperature when thinking), and hormonal analysis (Immordino-Yang & Gotlieb, 2017). Prior to these technologies, cognitive scientists relied on outcomes from tests with nonhuman animals (e.g., rats, monkeys, cats; Blakemore & Firth, 2005). While these studies gave researchers insight into how our brain functions and how emotions might be connected, the evidence was still removed from the human experience. Now, researchers are able to better theorize these connections. For example, researchers have discovered there are strong links between sensations that lead to empathy and activity in our brain stem. The brain stem is part of our affective networks and the very part of our brain that keeps us alive (Venkatraman et al., 2017; Immordino-Yang & Gotlieb, 2017). Using this example of the connection between the brain stem and empathy leads neuropsychologists to an understanding that biological survival (e.g., the brain stem) and sociocultural survival (e.g., the ability to connect with others) are intertwined (Immordino-Yang & Gotlieb, 2017). They are also able to better understand how disability can impact the affective networks in direct or indirect ways (Rose & Dalton, 2007).

For example, anxiety and depression can negatively affect a learner's motivation within a learning environment. More specifically, this could impact the learner's motivation to learn comprehension strategies. While motivation comes from within (intrinsic), it also comes from a learner's engagement with the goals, their engagement with the lesson, and how they are engaged by the teacher (Deci & Ryan, 2012: Palmer et al., 1994). A lower level of motivation means that the learner is entering the environment without the same opportunities as their peers (Rose & Dalton, 2007). Rather than looking at how disability affects the brain, though, the framework of UDL asks us to focus on the design of the learning environment and how that design can open opportunities for all learners to belong.

Returning to the case study at the beginning of the chapter, Dominique lowered the barriers linked to the principle of engagement by intentionally planning what she wanted them to experience. She wanted her learners to connect authentically to the poetry, whether reading or writing it. She wanted them to feel as though they would be able to read and write poetry with support. She wanted them to understand the work load, the amount of time they had, and how they could stay on the task. She offered a variety of poetry examples representing a diversity of style and comprehension difficulty. She placed them with reading partners and supported collaboration. She provided content-specific individualized feedback on their projects and writing. She made clear her expectations for quality products, but provided several pathways to achieve that level of quality. She made sure learners could identify ways to cope with writing setbacks and strategies to keep themselves on pace. And she provided them with tools to reflect on and monitor their own growth. These supports were offered to all of her learners, regardless of disability, ethnicity, language, or academic status. Each of these decisions were based on the principle of engagement, and each of these decisions were in place to help her learners move toward becoming purposeful and motivated.

Without opportunities to learn these socially valued skills, learners will continue to be at a disadvantage in developing satisfying adult lives, and professionals will have failed to fulfill the overarching purposes of education (Copeland & Cosbey, 2008). The argument for the meaningful inclusion of learners with IDD is clear, but the intersection with Carter's (this volume) work on belonging makes the argument stronger. When the learning environment is designed to only support a narrow set of learner traits (e.g., on-level reading proficiency or average to above average executive functioning skills), it is not an environment where all learners belong. Instead, the environment needs to be designed to support the full breadth of learner traits, so every learner can achieve the full sense of belonging.

4.4 Conclusion

This chapter was designed to guide the reader toward a deeper understanding of the UDL framework, specifically the principle of engagement and the affective networks, and to see how that information connects with the concepts of belonging and resilience. A discussion of the overall framework, with a tighter look at engagement, and the neuroscience of emotion provided the groundwork to look more closely at the case study of Dominique's classroom and see how an environment designed for all learners can provide a significant space for belonging and resilience.

While the UDL is a powerful framework, its impact on individuals with IDD is still not fully understood (Lowrey et al., 2017). The voices and experiences of learners with IDD are tantamount to understanding what impact the UDL can have on the sense of belonging and resilience. Without those voices, we cannot be sure these students are truly benefitting from the UDL in direct relation to belonging. We also do not have clarity around their growth in areas such as resilience. While there is clear intent woven into the framework to build an environment that incorporates belonging and resilience (e.g., foster collaboration and community), this has yet to be researched. Finally, teachers have been shown to struggle with understanding and implementing the principles of engagement (Capp, 2020), creating a potential gap in supporting students' connection to the environment. There is also a gap between teachers' implementation of the UDL and how they respond to students with IDD in those same environments (Lowrey et al., 2017; Rao et al., 2017). However, with the continued implementation and investigation of the UDL, the field of education with associated stakeholders (e.g., parents, community members) has the opportunity to position individuals with IDD to gain a stronger sense of belonging in inclusive environments as well as foster resilience while becoming purposeful, motivated, resourceful, knowledgeable, strategic, and goal-directed learners.

Questions for Thought and Discussion

1. How might an environment design like Domonique's affect the information shared by the educator with parents?
2. With a deeper understanding of how the affective networks are a part of each person's ability to learn, and understanding that we all instruct each other at times (e.g., how to put the dishes in the dishwasher, how to drive, how to install a door knob), in what ways does this alter how you will instruct others?
3. Articulate the parallel relationship between the social-ecological model of disability and the role of context in learning.
4. Evidence from the cognitive sciences offers proof of a deep connection between our social selves and our learning selves which lays the groundwork between belonging and learning. How might you represent this connection between belonging and learning through a graphic, a drawing, a poem, or some other artistic representation?

References

Agran, M., Cavin, M., Wehmeyer, M., & Palmer, S. (2006). Participation of students with moderate to severe disabilities in the general curriculum: The effects of the self-determined learning model of instruction. *Research and Practice for Persons with Severe Disabilities, 31*(3), 230–241. https://doi.org/10.1177/154079690603100303

Artiles, A. J. (2011). Toward an interdisciplinary understanding of educational equity and difference: The case of the racialization of ability. *Educational Researcher, 40*(9), 431–445. https://doi.org/10.3102/0013189X11429391

Blackburn, B. R. (2013). *Rigor is not a four-letter word*. Eye on Education.

Blakemore, S. J., & Firth, U. (2005). *The learning brain*. Blackwell.

Bronfenbrenner, U., & Morris, P. A. (1998). The ecology of developmental processes. *Handbook of Child Psychology, 1*(5), 993–1028.

Browder, D. M., Spooner, F., Ahlgrim-Delzell, L., Harris, A. A., & Wakemanxya, S. (2008). A meta-analysis on teaching mathematics to students with significant cognitive disabilities. *Exceptional Children, 74*(4), 407–432. https://doi.org/10.1177/001440290807400401

Capp, M. J. (2017). The effectiveness of universal design for learning: A meta-analysis of literature between 2013 and 2016. *International Journal of Inclusive Education, 21*(8), 791–807.

Capp, M. J. (2020). Teacher confidence to implement the principles, guidelines, and checkpoints of universal design for learning. *International Journal of Inclusive Education, 24*(7), 706–720. https://doi.org/10.1080/13603116.2018.1482014

CAST. (2018). *Universal design for learning guidelines version 2.2 [graphic organizer]*. Author.

Carter, E. W. (2016). A place of belonging: Research at the intersection of faith and disability. *Review & Expositor, 113*(2), 167–180.

Carter, E. W. (this volume). Dimensions of belonging for individuals with intellectual and developmental disabilities. In J. L. Jones & K. L. Gallus (Vol. Eds.), *Belonging and resilience in individuals with intellectual and developmental disabilities – Community and family engagement*. Springer.

Cohen, G. L., Garcia, J., Apfel, N., & Master, A. (2006). Reducing the racial achievement gap: A social-psychological intervention. *Science, 313*(5791), 1307–1310. https://doi.org/10.1126/science.1128317

Copeland, S. R., & Cosbey, J. (2008). Making progress in the general curriculum: Rethinking effective instructional practices. *Research and Practice for Persons with Severe Disabilities, 34*(1), 214–227. https://doi.org/10.2511/rpsd.33.4.214

Coyne, P., Evans, M., & Karger, J. (2017). Use of a UDL literacy environment by middle school students with intellectual and developmental disabilities. *Intellectual and Developmental Disabilities, 55*(1), 4–14. https://doi.org/10.1352/1934-9556-55.1.4

Damasio, A. D. (1994). *Descartes' error: Emotion, reason, and the human brain*. Putnam.

Deci, E. L., & Ryan, R. M. (2012). Motivation, personality, and development within embedded social contexts: An overview of self-determination theory. In R. M. Ryan (Ed.), *Oxford library of psychology. The Oxford handbook of human motivation* (pp. 85–107). Oxford University Press.

Dymond, S. K., Renzaglia, A., Rosenstein, A., Chun, E. J., Banks, R. A., Niswander, V., & Gilson, C. L. (2006). Using a participatory action research approach to create a universally designed inclusive high school science course: A case study. *Research and Practice for Persons with Severe Disabilities, 31*(4), 293–308. https://doi.org/10.1177/154079690603100403

Gregg, N. (2012). Increasing access to learning for the adult basic education learner with learning disabilities: Evidence-based accommodation research. *Journal of Learning Disabilities, 45*(1), 47–63. https://doi.org/10.1177/0022219411426855

Hammer, T., Crethar, H., & Cannon, K. (2016). Convergence of identities through the lens of relational-cultural theory. *Journal of Creativity in Mental Health, 11*(2), 126–141. https://doi.org/10.1080/15401383.2016.1181596

Hamre, B. K., & Pianta, R. C. (2001). Early teacher–child relationships and the trajectory of children's school outcomes through eighth grade. *Child Development, 72*(2), 625–638. https://doi.org/10.1111/1467-8624.00301

Immordino-Yang, M. H. (2007). A tale of two cases: Lessons for education from the study of two boys living with half their brains. Mind, Brain, and Education, 1(2), 66–83.

Immordino-Yang, M. H., & Gotlieb, R. (2017). Embodied brains, social minds, cultural meaning: Integrating neuroscientific and educational research on socialaffective development. American Educational Research Journal, 54(1_suppl), 344S–367S.

Immordino-Yang, M. H., & Damasio, A. (2011). We feel, therefore we learn: The relevance of affective and neuroscience in education. *LEARNing Landscapes, 5*(1), 115–130. https://doi.org/10.36510/learnland.v5i1.535

Immordino-Yang, M. H., & Gotlieb, R. (2017). Embodied brains, social minds, cultural meaning: Integrating neuroscientific and educational research on social-affective development. *American Educational Research Journal, 54*(1), 344S–367S. https://doi.org/10.3102/0002831216669780

Johnston, P. H. (2004). *Choice words: How our language affects children's learning*. Stenhouse.

Jorgensen, C. M., McSheehan, M., & Sonnenmeier, R. M. (2007). Presumed competence reflected in the educational programs of students with IDD before and after the Beyond Access professional development intervention. *Journal of Intellectual & Developmental Disability, 32*(4), 248–262. https://doi.org/10.1080/13668250701704238

Lane, R. D., & Nadel, L. (2000). *Cognitive neuroscience of emotion*. Oxford University Press.

Ledoux, J. (2003). *Synaptic self: How our brains become who we are*. Penguin.

Levykh, M. G. (2008). The affective establishment and maintenance of Vygotsky's zone of proximal development. *Educational Theory, 58*(1), 83–101. https://doi.org/10.1111/j.1741-5446.2007.00277.x

Lieber, J., Horn, E., Palmer, S., & Fleming, K. (2008). Access to the general education curriculum for preschoolers with disabilities: Children's school success. *Exceptionality, 16*(1), 18–32. https://doi.org/10.1080/09362830701796776

Lowrey, K. A., Hollingshead, A., Howery, K., & Bishop, J. B. (2017). More than one way: Stories of UDL and inclusive classrooms. *Research and Practice for Persons with Severe Disabilities, 42*(4), 225–242. https://doi.org/10.1177/1540796917711668

Meyer, A., Rose, D. H., & Gordon, D. (2014). *Universal design for learning: Theory and practice*. CAST Publishing.

Mitchell, D. (2014). *What really works in special and inclusive education: Using evidence-based teaching strategies*. Routledge.

Morales, R., & Macpherson, F. (2017, July). All is vanity. In F. Macpherson (Ed.), *The illusions index*. Retrieved from https://www.illusionsindex.org/i/all-is-vanity.

Nasir, N. I. S. (2012). *Racialized identities: Race and achievement from African American youth*. Stanford University Press.

Nelson, L. L. (2019). *A tree for all: Your coloring book of UDL principles and practice*. CAST.

Nelson, L. L. (2021). *Design and deliver: Planning and teaching using universal design for learning* (2nd ed.). Paul H. Brookes.

Palmer, B. M., Codling, R. M., & Gambrel, L. B. (1994). In their own words: What elementary students have to say about motivation to read. *The Reading Teacher, 48*, 176–178.

Panksepp, J. (1998). *Affective neuroscience*. Oxford University Press.

Peets, K. (2009). The effects of context on the classroom discourse skills of children with language impairment. *Language, Speech & Hearing Services in Schools, 40*(1), 5–16. https://doi.org/10.1044/0161-1461(2008/07-0012

Rao, K., Smith, S. J., & Lowrey, K. A. (2017). UDL and intellectual disability: What do we know and where do we go? *Intellectual and Developmental Disabilities, 55*(1), 37–47. https://doi.org/10.1352/1934-9556-55.1.37

Rose, D. H. (2011). *Acknowledging learner variability: Changes in UDL guidelines 2.0.* https://www.youtube.com/watch?v=rlv6JJQOz64.

Rose, D. H., & Dalton, B. (2007). *Plato revisited: Learning through listening in the digital world.* CAST, Inc. Retrieved from http://citeseerx.ist.psu.edu/viewdoc/download;jsessionid=F4434F5D53B397CD7B115066D5E750B3?doi=10.1.1.112.3313&rep=rep1&type=pdf

Rose, D. H., & Meyer, A. (2002). *Teaching every student in the digital age*. ASCD.

Rose, D. H., & Strangman, N. (2007). Universal Design for Learning: Meeting the challenge of individual learning differences through a neurocognitive perspective. *Universal Access in the Information Society, 5*(4), 381–391. https://doi.org/10.1007/s10209-006-0062-8

Shogren, K. A. (2013). A social–ecological analysis of the self-determination literature. *Mental Retardation, 51*(6), 496–511. https://doi.org/10.1352/1934-9556-51.6.496

Shogren, K. A., Faggella-Luby, M. N., Bae, S. J., & Wehmeyer, M. L. (2004). The effect of choice-making as an intervention for problem behavior: A meta-analysis. *Journal of Positive Behavior Interventions, 6*(4), 228–237. https://doi.org/10.1177/10983007040060040401

Steele, C. M., & Aronson, J. (1995). Stereotype threat and the intellectual test performance of African Americans. *Journal of Personality and Social Psychology, 69*, 797–811. https://doi.org/10.1037/0022-3514.69.5.797

Venkatraman, A., Edlow, B. L., & Immordino-Yang, M. H. (2017). The brainstem in emotion: A review. *Frontiers in Neuroanatomy, 11*, 15.

Vygotsky, L. S., Hanfmann, E., & Vakar, G. (1962). *Thought and language*. MIT Press.

Wang, M., Haertel, G., & Walberg, H. (1998). *Building educational resilience*. Phi Delta Kappa Educational Foundation.

Whitted, K. S. (2011). Understanding how social and emotional skill deficits contribute to school failure. *Preventing School Failure: Alternative Education for Children and Youth, 55*(1), 10–16. https://doi.org/10.1080/10459880903286755

Chapter 5
Mental Health and Developmental Disabilities: Fostering Belonging and Resilience for Individuals and Families

Emily Tucker, Karyn Harvey, Kami L. Gallus, and Jennifer L. Jones

Disparities in the mental health of individuals with intellectual and developmental disabilities (IDD) have been observed for centuries. Prevalence estimates suggest that 30–50% of individuals with IDD experience at least one mental health disorder (Cooper et al., 2007; Munir, 2016). Common mental health disorders among individuals with IDD include mood disorders, anxiety disorders, and impulse control disorders (Stavrakaki & Lunsky, 2007). For individuals with IDD, mental health needs often introduce additional challenges in daily life, further impacting belonging and resilience for an already marginalized and stigmatized population. Despite experiencing consistently higher prevalence rates of mental health diagnoses, individuals with IDD also experience significant barriers to accessing mental health care, constituting what Krahn et al. (2006) termed a "cascade of disparities" (p. 71). Among the common barriers to accessing mental health care for individuals with IDD are the availability and affordability of care (Douma et al., 2006; Krauss et al., 2003). As a result of ongoing inequities in mental health, the holistic, biopsychosocial well-being of many individuals with IDD, as well as their family members, is often ignored, overlooked, and unaddressed.

The current chapter aims to highlight the role of mental health in fostering belonging and resilience in individuals with IDD and their families. The chapter begins by examining how the separation of the professional fields of mental health and developmental disabilities perpetuates ongoing disparities resulting from the

E. Tucker
East Carolina University, Greenville, NC, USA

K. Harvey
Park Ave Group, Baltimore, MD, USA

K. L. Gallus (✉) · J. L. Jones
Oklahoma State University, Stillwater, OK, USA
e-mail: kami.gallus@okstate.edu

J. L. Jones, K. L. Gallus (eds.), *Belonging and Resilience in Individuals with Developmental Disabilities*, Emerging Issues in Family and Individual Resilience, https://doi.org/10.1007/978-3-030-81277-5_5

underdiagnosis and misdiagnosis of mental health disorders, as well as the exclusion of many individuals with IDD from mental health care. Noting the impact of inequities in mental health and mental health care on belonging and resilience of individuals with IDD, the chapter calls professionals across diverse fields of study to consider a systemic and holistic perspective of supports and services that includes increased attention to the mental health needs and improved access to adequate mental health care for individuals with IDD.

5.1 Mental Health and Developmental Disabilities

Despite the current identification of mental health and developmental disabilities as two distinct fields of specialized knowledge and practice, the two professional disciplines share a great deal of history and evolution. During much of the twentieth century, the primary model of care for individuals with chronic mental health and/or IDD, previously referred to as "the mentally ill and handicapped," involved congregate care in institutional settings. At the time, institutions, in which "patients" lived and were treated by professional staff, were considered the most moral and effective way to care for individuals with severe cognitive and mental impairments (Wehmeyer, 2013). In spite of these ideals, the institutional model of care pushed people with severe mental health disorders and/or IDD further to the margins, excluding them from daily life in most communities.

In the late twentieth century, the deinstitutionalization movement arose amidst the era of the civil rights movement when many marginalized groups were being incorporated into mainstream society. Among other forces, the evidence that isolated living in institutions often led to treatment that was cruel and inhumane drove the deinstitutionalization movement for individuals with severe mental health disorders and/or IDD. While advocacy for the rights of individuals with mental health disorders and IDD began with the voices of family members and loved ones, gradually, individuals and families were joined and supported by a range of professionals, organizations, associations, and some governmental agencies. While the advocacy efforts of professionals were initially united by a shared focus on ensuring the deinstitutionalization of all individuals, overtime the professional organizations, associations, and governmental agencies grew more and more distinct as efforts shifted to advocating for and meeting the unique needs based either on one's mental health or disability—thus forming the foundation of the two distinct service fields of mental health and developmental disabilities often recognized today.

With the closing of institutions, the responsibility for the provision of health services for individuals with severe mental health disorders and IDD was transferred from the institutions to less isolating community-based services. Though the goal of deinstitutionalization—improving treatment and the quality of life of individuals—is known best practice, the separation of community-based services accentuated the polarized conceptualizations of mental health and IDD as two mutually exclusive service systems with two separate groups of service recipients

(Pickard & Akinsola, 2010). The distinction between professionals and services across the two fields of mental health and developmental disabilities has become more prominent over time as ongoing advocacy efforts focus on developing and implementing effective, community-based systems of care. The polarization of the two fields has resulted in professionals from both sides of the gap often feeling ill-equipped to fully address the mental health support needs of individuals with IDD (Hronis et al., 2018). Decades into the deinstitutionalization movement, the complexities of community-based services continue to challenge professionals across both fields. Despite the hopes of many who advocated for deinstitutionalization, simply changing the living location from large congregate care settings to living in the community has proven to be an inadequate substitute for effective mental health care for individuals with IDD (Pickard & Akinsola, 2010).

5.1.1 Diagnostic Overshadowing

The stigma associated with historical models of institutional care, as well as the splintering of the two fields, undoubtedly continues to impact the distorted views of the mental health needs that contribute to ongoing disparities in the mental health care of individuals with IDD. Professionals across both fields have often viewed individuals with IDD as incapable of developing psychopathology (Reiss et al., 1982; Sovner & Hurley, 1983). Historically, when internalizing or externalizing behaviors (e.g., physical assault, self-injurious behavior) were noted, such behaviors were attributed to limitations in cognition and communication rather than the possible presence of mental health symptoms (Gardner & Cole, 1990; Szymanski & Grossman, 1984), a phenomenon often referred to as *diagnostic overshadowing* (Reiss et al., 1982). For instance, behaviors such as skin picking are often understood as a symptom of IDD, rather than as a symptom of an anxiety disorder. The ongoing practice of predominantly attributing symptoms and behaviors to an individual's disability often limits the exploration of the possibility of mental health symptoms, thus perpetuating the myth that individuals with IDD are incapable of developing psychopathology and consequently reinforcing their exclusion from mental health care (Pickard & Akinsola, 2010; Reiss et al., 1982).

The phenomenon of diagnostic overshadowing highlights the stigma as well as the lack of awareness and training surrounding the mental health needs of individuals with IDD. Within current models of supports and services, when an individual is given a diagnosis of intellectual disability, the label of disability frequently overshadows other basic, ordinary human needs. As a result, individuals with IDD are often stripped of the dignity of recognition of their mental health and consequent need for and right to mental health care. Failure to offer competent community-based mental health care communicates to an already marginalized population that their mental health and well-being is not valued—that they do not belong in the therapy room. To establish and sustain an identity of belonging, professionals across both fields must begin to acknowledge, understand, and value the mental health needs of individuals with IDD.

5.2 The Story of John

Throughout the last 34 years of my (KH's) career as a licensed psychologist, my greatest teachers have been the numerous clients with IDD I have been privileged to work alongside. One of my most memorable teachers along the way was a young man named John.[1] John was born addicted to cocaine. In addition to being weaned off the drug in a neonatal unit, he suffered numerous other medical complications requiring surgeries and other interventions. His birthmother made sporadic visits to the hospital during his first 2 months of life, but eventually relocated with no forwarding address. Due to his complex medical support needs, John was unable to transition into foster care. At just 2 months of age, John was alone. He remained in the hospital for over 2 years until he was adopted by a warm and caring family. John's adoptive mother was highly aware of his support needs, including the biological effects of his in utero cocaine exposure. As John grew older, it became apparent; he needed support with executive functioning, related to his diagnoses of impulse control disorder (American Psychiatric Association, 2013) and attention deficit hyperactive disorder (ADHD; American Psychiatric Association, 2013). Once John started school, he was diagnosed with intellectual disability and placed in segregated special education classrooms. When John was in elementary school, his adoptive father died of cancer. While John's older, adoptive siblings were devastated by the loss, it seemed they were able to effectively grieve the loss of their father and carry on with their lives. As John grew, the negative outcomes of his attachment injuries and emotional support needs intensified. Instead of getting the support he needed, John was labeled a "behavior problem" in the school system. He was eventually removed from his public school setting and in middle school was transferred to an out-of-state residential school. Having lost his birthmother and his adoptive father, and now removed from his family and support system, John found himself alone once again.

At school, John's externalized behaviors increased and eventually escalated to property destruction. After each episode of destruction, John would cry and apologize—repeatedly declaring, "I don't know why I did it. I'm sorry." When John aged out of the education system at 21, he was transferred back to his state of origin and received state-funded services. Within his state-funded services system, John was once again labeled a behavior problem. John worked to meet his own emotional support needs by trying to ask for help when he felt overwhelmed. He tried to talk with the direct support professionals (DSPs) in his group home but felt they ignored him or were too busy to talk. During this same time, John developed a relationship

[1] John is a pseudonym used to maintain confidentiality.

with a young woman, Sally, who he met at a day program. In Sally, John found a partner he was able to talk to and confide in. As a result, John felt better, and his DSP reported a significant decrease in John's negative behaviors. However, when his relationship with Sally ended, John felt alone once more. When he tried to talk about his feelings with his staff and other service providers, John felt ignored. With no one to talk to, John's emotional support needs became too great for him to carry alone. One night, John went to his room and set his trash can on fire. The fire accidentally spread to John's bedroom curtains, and before long the flames engulfed his home. Thankfully, John, the DSP, and his housemates managed to safely evacuate. As a result of the fire, John was arrested and incarcerated. While incarcerated, John was labeled an arsonist and referred to a program for people with IDD and forensic involvement.

After John completed his time in incarceration, he was court ordered to be placed in an alternative residential program with an intensive behavioral plan. Five years later, I (KH) met John for the first time when he began individual counseling. Through our work together, John began to acknowledge and address his early life trauma and loss. Through his work in counseling, John developed a strong sense of identity. This strong identity allowed John to develop the skills he needed to advocate for his support needs more effectively. With the help of his staff, John began looking for a job and for a new home with roommates he liked and DSPs with whom he felt safe. John continues to experience difficult days and hard times, but he has learned to engage with staff and reach out to friends when he needs support. Shedding the former labels of "behavior problem" and "arsonist," John now refers to himself as a "proud black, gay man." He enjoys volunteering at various organizations and continues to look for a job.

John's story illustrates how the mental health needs of individuals with IDD are all too often misunderstood and/or unaddressed, leading to a lack of opportunities for belonging. John did not belong to his biological family. He did not belong in school with his peers. Eventually, due to his externalized behaviors, John did not even belong in community-based residential services. Fortunately, after many years of searching, John was able to find the mental health supports he needed to strong sense of identity—an identity of belonging that fostered resilience.

5.3 Belonging, Resilience, and Mental Health

There is much to be learned from John's story. Our combined years of experience across the two fields of mental health and developmental disabilities have taught us that many individuals with IDD have similar experiences of grief, loss, stress, or crisis. Still, the mental health symptoms and needs commonly associated with these experiences often remain overlooked or unaddressed in the shadow of the IDD label. As highlighted in John's experience, when individuals with IDD display mental health symptoms, those symptoms are often mislabeled as behavioral problems and treated with increased medications, segregation, and/or behavioral restrictions.

Unfortunately, John's experience of receiving adequate mental health support, albeit much later than he needed, remains the exception rather than the norm for most individuals with IDD. This is particularly concerning when considering how critical positive mental health and adequate mental health care are to the capacity of individuals with IDD to pursue interests and activities that enhance belonging and resilience. Positive mental health is characterized by a person's ability to fulfill a number of key daily functions and activities, including the ability to cope with normal life stressors, express and manage a range of positive and negative emotions, and the ability to form and maintain relationships and work productively to contribute to one's community. Further, there is strong evidence that belonging, in particular, is related to positive mental health within the general public (Greenaway et al., 2015; Khan et al., 2014; Sani et al., 2012). In mental health terms, one's sense of belonging refers to the experience of feeling valued and the perception of fit or connectedness within one's system or environment (Hagerty & Patusky, 1995). A strong sense of belonging has been associated with less severe depression across various populations of individuals without disabilities (Chassin et al., 2004; Choenarom et al., 2005; Sangon, 2004; Turner & McLaren, 2011). One's sense of belonging also has been proposed as a key factor associated with resilience. Resilience refers to the capacity to cope successfully with significant adversity or risk and has long been a subject of interest in the field of mental health.

Professionals across diverse fields can and should play a significant role in facilitating belonging and fostering resilience for individuals with IDD. According to Carter (this volume, Chap. 2), for individuals with IDD and their families to experience true belonging that fosters resilience, the following ten dimensions must be salient in daily life, to be (a) present, (b) invited, (c) welcomed, (d) known, (e) accepted, (f) supported, (g) heard, (h) befriended, (i) needed, and (j) loved. Beyond simply ensuring that individuals experience each of the ten dimensions of belonging within the context of the community-based supports and services they provide, professionals across the fields of mental health and developmental disabilities should work to support individuals with IDD to develop an identity of belonging across multiple contexts. An "identity of belonging" validates that individuals with IDD belong in communities and, similar to peers without disabilities, require both formal and natural supports in managing life's stressors, navigating relationships, and enhancing mental health.

5.3.1 The Biopsychosocial Framework of Mental Health

John's story above illustrates the disparities that are perpetuated when the fields of mental health and developmental disabilities remain siloed, and the medical model of disability (See Jones & Gallus, Chap. 1, this volume) remains a dominant mental model used by professionals. In contrast to the reductionistic, medical model of mental health, Engel's biopsychosocial framework (1980, 1997) offers a holistic approach to mental health and wellness that conceptualizes individuals as simultaneously biological, psychological, and social beings. Compared to the medical model, which reduces the focus of mental health and well-being to the physical or biological factors of the individual (i.e., disability), the biopsychosocial framework aligns with both the multidimensional framework and social-ecological approach of disability (Buntinx & Schalock, 2010) by highlighting the complexity of individual factors associated with mental health. Thus, mental health care must be expanded to address the biological, psychological, and social needs of individuals with IDD in an integrated manner. While professionals in the field of developmental disabilities have historically been tasked with addressing the basic or biological needs of individuals with IDD (e.g., food, shelter, medication, physical health care), mental health professionals have historically been tasked with meeting the psychosocial needs (e.g., treating mental health symptoms, promoting healthy relationships). The biopsychosocial framework suggests that to effectively support and meet the mental health needs of individuals with IDD, professionals must be equipped to acknowledge and address the complex interaction among biological, psychological, and social needs.

5.3.2 A Holistic Approach: Coexistence of Intellectual and Developmental Disabilities and Mental Health

A holistic view of the complex systems and interactions that impact individuals with IDD requires a multidisciplinary team approach. While there will always be a need for the two distinct, professional fields of mental health and developmental disabilities, a systemic model requires the fields to work together to bridge the gap in mental health care for individuals with IDD. However, when professionals across the fields of mental health and developmental disabilities adopt a biopsychosocial framework that acknowledges the holistic needs of individuals with IDD, those same professionals often grapple with questions concerning the provision of systemic supports and services. Many of the current constraints are consequences of professional uncertainties (e.g., Who is qualified to provide support? What practices offer the best support?). These uncertainties continue to perpetuate the inequities in mental health care. At the crux of the inequities is the ongoing argument of whether working with clients with IDD should be seen as a specialty for a few or a general competency for all licensed mental health professionals—leaving many individuals with IDD and their families struggling to access mental health care.

For individuals with IDD, this inequity is not evidenced solely in mental health care but is an all-too-familiar disparity that individuals and their family members experience across multiple systems and throughout the lifespan. As noted in several chapters within this volume, reductionistic thinking has led to the ongoing segregation of individuals with IDD across multiple community contexts—all of which are known to impact mental health. Until professionals across all fields of study, not just mental health, recognize and advocate that individuals with IDD belong in our communities—where we live, work, worship, learn, and play—the inequities that threaten individual, family, and community resilience will remain.

By working together across fields and acknowledging individuals with IDD as the experts of their own mental health, professionals can improve the outcomes for individuals with IDD and their families. Beart et al. (2005) offered that for individuals without IDD, the understanding of disability will always lie at the level of discourse rather than that of experience. They challenged researchers to acknowledge their limited perspective and to "try to understand at the level of experience by listening carefully to the people who live this identity every day" (Beart et al., 2005, p. 55). We pose this is not only a challenge for the researcher, but for all professionals working alongside individuals with IDD and their families. In keeping with the professional responsibility to develop cultural competence in working with diverse populations, individuals with IDD and their families represent an underserved and marginalized population that all professionals must seek to better understand and effectively support.

The mental models we as professionals bring to our scholarship and practice greatly impact our work. Thus, it is vital for professionals to identify and acknowledge their personal values and beliefs regarding the coexistence of IDD and mental health. As professionals, our working mental models determine not only the terminology we use but also provide the basis upon which we devise strategies for providing supports and services. When we understand disability as a natural part of human diversity, rather than a medical condition that needs to be cured or fixed, then the development of cultural competence that includes individuals with IDD becomes the ethical obligation of all professionals rather than the responsibility of a few with specialized training.

For the growing number of licensed mental health professionals who desire to effectively support the mental health needs of individuals with IDD, the current lack of training and resources poses a challenge, and many who wish to offer support feel unqualified (Hronis et al., 2018). Nonetheless, despite the dearth of clinical and empirical knowledge regarding the mental health needs and care of individuals with IDD, licensed mental health professionals remain the most qualified professionals to address the unmet mental health needs for all populations. Embracing/utilizing mental models within the mental health field to understand and respond to disability as a natural part of human diversity and thus as a component of cultural competence highlights a key skill set of most licensed mental health professionals who are highly trained and well-equipped to facilitate connection with clients across diverse backgrounds. It is important to remember that cultural competence represents more than a professional skill set; it is a professional's personal and ongoing desire and commitment to use those skills to understand diverse client experiences. While more research on the mental health needs of individuals with IDD and their families is certainly needed to advance training of professionals to provide culturally informed mental health care for individuals with IDD, the unmet mental health care needs facing individuals with IDD and their families simply cannot wait for research and education to catch up. Licensed mental health professionals who are willing to answer the current call to provide mental health care alongside individuals with IDD and their family members is key to advancing mental health services and addressing the ongoing disparities many individuals and their families face. Expanding diversity perspectives within mental health to include attunement to disability is an important first step in promoting licensed mental health professionals who feel equipped and qualified to provide effective mental health care that meets the needs of individuals with IDD. Resources for professionals working to support the mental health needs of individuals with IDD are included at the end of in this chapter.

5.4 Conclusion

Experience has taught us that even John's story of eventually finding the mental health supports he needed remains an exception, rather than the norm for individuals with IDD in need of community-based mental health services. Perhaps some of the challenges John faced could have been avoided if his mental health needs had been acknowledged and validated at an earlier age and adequate mental health care had been accessible. Positive mental health is critical to the capacity of people, including individuals with IDD, to pursue interests and activities that enhance belonging and overall quality of life. Applying a holistic, biopsychosocial framework enhances the quality of mental health care of individuals with IDD. We hope this chapter serves as a call to engagement for all professionals to begin or continue working toward an expanded, biopsychosocial framework to supports and services that enhances the positive mental health and resilience of all. As professionals across fields work to bridge the gap in mental health care, true belonging can be fostered that promotes resilience for individuals, families, and communities. In turn, when individuals with IDD begin to fully experience belonging and resilience, the cascade of mental health disparities can begin to be addressed.

Resources for Professionals Supporting Mental Health Needs of Individuals with Intellectual and Developmental Disabilities and Families
Workbooks

- Dr. Karyn Harvey compiled a library of free workbooks to help guide professionals supporting individuals in healing after a wide range of life challenges. https://karynharvey.org/about.html
- The *Strong Minds Activity Guide* is a free workbook published by Special Olympics: Strong Minds providing accessible visuals and specific coping strategies to help manage stress. https://media.specialolympics.org/resources/health/disciplines/strongminds/Strong-Minds-YA-Activity-Cards-08-2020.pdf?_ga=2.237808648.904192511.1615567812-999014929.1615567812

Resource Books

- *Positive Identity Development: An Alternative Treatment Approach for Individuals with Mild and Moderate Intellectual Disabilities* provides a theoretical framework and specific techniques professionals can use to support individuals with IDD in fostering an identity of belonging.
- *Trauma-Informed Behavioral Interventions: What Works and What Doesn't* offers a mental health-focused framework for effective supports and techniques.
- *Trauma and Healing in the Lives of People with Intellectual Disability* combines Dr. Harvey's years of experience focused specifically on supporting individuals experiences mental health symptoms related to trauma.

Professional Organizations

- The American Association on Intellectual and Developmental Disabilities (AAIDD), the oldest and largest interdisciplinary organization for professional and others concerned about IDD. AAIDD posts resources and research on their website regarding the mental health of individuals with IDD. https://www.aaidd.org/intellectual-disability/intersectionality/idd-mental-health#.YEt_FGhKhA9
- The National Association for the Dually Diagnosed (NADD) is leading the way in education, consultation, and training related to community-based, whole-person treatment for the mental health needs of those with IDD. NADD hosts annual conferences, publishes up-to-date research, and supports mental health professionals in providing quality mental health supports. https://www.thenadd.org

Questions for Thought and Discussion

1. How would applying a biopsychosocial framework impact your scholarship and/or practice alongside individuals with intellectual and developmental disabilities and their families?
2. What steps can you take to enhance belonging for individuals with intellectual and developmental disabilities in mental health care?
3. How can the fields of mental health and developmental disabilities work together to enhance belonging and resilience for individuals with intellectual and developmental disabilities and their families?

References

American Psychiatric Association. (2013). *Diagnostic and statistical manual of mental disorders* (5th ed.). American Psychiatric Publishing.

Beart, S., Hardy, G., & Buchan, L. (2005). How people with intellectual disabilities view their social identity: A review of the literature. *Journal of Applied Research in Intellectual Disabilities, 18*, 47–56. https://doi.org/10.1111/j.1468-3148.2004.00218.x

Buntinx, W., & Schalock, R. (2010). Models of disability, quality of life, and individualized supports: Implications for professional practice in intellectual disability. *Journal of Policy and Practice in Intellectual Disabilities, 7*, 283–294. https://doi.org/10.1111/j.1741-1130.2010.00278.x

Carter, E. W. (this volume). Dimensions of belonging for individuals with intellectual and developmental disabilities. In J. Jones & K. Gallus (Vol. Eds.), *Belonging and resilience in individuals with intellectual and developmental disabilities – Community and family engagement.* Springer.

Chassin, L., Carle, A. C., Nissim-Sabat, D., & Kumpfer, K. L. (2004). Fostering resilience in children of alcoholic parents. In K. I. Maton, C. J. Schellenbach, B. J. Leadbeater, & A. L. Solarz (Eds.), *Investing in children, youth, families, and communities: Strengths-based research and policy* (pp. 137–155). American Psychological Association. https://doi.org/10.1037/10660-008

Choenarom, C., Williams, R., & Hagerty, B. (2005). The role of sense of belonging and social support on stress and depression in individuals with depression. *Archives of Psychiatric Nursing, 19*, 18–29. https://doi.org/10.1016/j.apnu.2004.11.003

Cooper, S. A., Smiley, E., Morrinson, J., Williamson, A., & Allan, L. (2007). Mental ill-health in adults with intellectual disabilities: Prevalence and associated factors. *British Journal of Psychiatry, 190*, 27–35. https://doi.org/10.1192/bjp.bp.106.022483

Douma, J., Dekker, M., & Koot, H. (2006). Supporting parents of youths with intellectual disabilities and psychopathology. *Journal of Intellectual Disability Research, 50*, 570–581. https://doi.org/10.1111/j.1365-2788.2006.00825.x

Engel, G. L. (1980). The clinical applications of the biopsychosocial model. *American Journal of Psychiatry, 137*, 535–544. https://doi.org/10.1176/ajp.137.5.535

Engel, G. L. (1997). The need for a new medical model: A challenge for biomedicine. *Science, 196*, 129–136. https://doi.org/10.1126/science.847460

Gardner, W., & Cole, C. (1990). Aggression and related conduct difficulties. In J. L. Matson (Ed.), *Handbook of behavior modification with the mentally retarded* (pp. 225–251). Springer. https://doi.org/10.1007/978-1-4899-2501-5_9

Greenaway, K., Cruwys, T., Haslam, S., & Jetten, J. (2015). Social identities promote well-being because they satisfy global psychological needs. *European Journal of Social Psychology, 46*, 294–307. https://doi.org/10.1002/ejsp.2169

Hagerty, B., & Patusky, K. (1995). Developing a measure of sense of belonging. *Nursing Research, 44*, 9–13. https://doi.org/10.1097/00006199-199501000-00003

Hronis, A., Roberts, L., & Kneebone, I. (2018). Assessing the confidence of Australian mental health practitioners in delivering therapy to people with intellectual disability. *Intellectual and Developmental Disabilities, 56*, 202–211. https://doi.org/10.1352/1934-9556-56.3.202

Khan, S., Hopkins, N., Tewari, S., Srinivasan, N., Reicher, S., & Ozakinci, G. (2014). Efficacy and well-being in rural north India: The role of social identification with a large-scale community identity. *European Journal of Social Psychology, 44*, 787–798. https://doi.org/10.1002/ejsp.2060

Krahn, G., Hammond, L., & Turner, A. (2006). A cascade of disparities: Health and health care access for people with intellectual disabilities. *Mental Retardation and Developmental Disabilities Research Reviews, 12*, 70–82. https://doi.org/10.1002/mrdd.20098

Krauss, M., Gulley, S., Sciegaj, M., Wells, N., & Taylor, S. (2003). Access to specialty medical care for children with mental retardation, Autism, and other special health care needs. *Intellectual and Developmental Disabilities, 42*, 329–339. https://doi.org/10.1352/0047-6765(2003)41<329:ATSMCF>2.0.CO;2

Munir, K. M. (2016). The co-occurrence of mental disorders in children and adolescents with intellectual disability/intellectual developmental disorder. *Current Opinion in Psychiatry, 29*, 95–102. https://doi.org/10.1097/YCO.0000000000000236

Pickard, M., & Akinsola, T. (2010). The association between psychopathology and intellectual disability. In N. Bouras & G. Holt (Eds.), *Mental health services for adults with intellectual disability: Strategies and solutions* (pp. 101–114). Psychology Press. https://doi.org/10.4324/9780203856086-15

Reiss, S., Levitan, G. W., & Szyszko, J. (1982). Emotional disturbance and mental retardation: Diagnostic overshadowing. *American Journal of Mental Deficiency, 86*, 567–574.

Sangon, S. (2004). Predictors of depression in Thai women. *Research and Theory for Nursing Practice, 18*, 243–260. https://doi.org/10.1891/rtnp.18.2.243.61276

Sani, F., Herrera, M., Wakefield, J., Boroch, O., & Gulyas, C. (2012). Comparing social contact and group identification as predictors of mental health. *British Journal of Social Psychology, 51*, 781–790. https://doi.org/10.1111/j.2044-8309.2012.02101.x

Sovner, R., & Hurley, A. (1983). Do the mentally retarded suffer from affective illness? *Archives of General Psychiatry, 40*, 61–67. https://doi.org/10.1001/archpsyc.1983.01790010063008

Stavrakaki, C., & Lunsky, Y. (2007). Depression, anxiety and adjustment disorders in people with intellectual disabilities. In N. Bouras & G. Holt (Eds.), *Psychiatric and behavioral disorders in intellectual and developmental disabilities* (pp. 113–130). Cambridge University Press.

Szymanski, L., & Grossman, H. (1984). Dual implications of "dual diagnosis": Guest editorial. *Mental Retardation, 22*(4), 155–156.

Turner, L., & McLaren, S. (2011). Social support and sense of belonging as protective factors in the rumination–depressive symptoms relation among Australian women. *Women & Health, 51*, 151–167. https://doi.org/10.1080/03630242.2011.558004

Wehmeyer, M. (2013). *The story of intellectual disability: An evolution of meaning, understanding, and public perception*. Brookes.

Chapter 6
Whose Am I? Spiritual Pathways Into the Heart of Belonging

Bill Gaventa

In 1975, my first full-time job was the Protestant chaplain at one of the old hellacious institutions in upstate New York. In my office, I found a copy of a 1950s Family Manual given to families when a child or family member was admitted. Based on the ubiquitous professional and social consensus that the institution was where their children "belonged," the manual suggested that, once admitted, families were not to come visit for at least 6 months to give their sons and daughters, brothers and sisters, "time to settle in"—to become institutionalized. For new residents of the institution, belonging, the spiritual question of "Whose we are?", was no longer answered by one's relationships, but by one's place, apart from community, in other words, "Where do they belong?"

Less than a month into the job, two core spiritual needs emerged as the primary concerns of my congregation: celebration and belonging. First, how could pastoral care and religious services, along with other disciplines, enable the people living at that institution to feel their lives had value—that they were celebrated, rather than stigmatized? Within my Christian faith, worship services and pastoral care that focused on God's love for them was a start, but I sometimes felt like an idealistic Don Quixote tilting at windmills. Second, in the face of the tragedy of separation and isolation, was it even possible to help the people in my congregation feel they belonged to a wider community, including the communities of the people of God?

Conversations about the sacredness of life and belonging have been ongoing for thousands of years among faith communities and across theological traditions. When related to people with disabilities, the conversations have included both wonderful and harmful discussions regarding not only their place in faith communities but in the kingdom of God, however defined. In the last century, as the focus of ministry with people with intellectual and developmental disabilities (IDD) moved,

B. Gaventa (✉)
Institute on Theology and Disability, Austin, TX, USA

J. L. Jones, K. L. Gallus (eds.), *Belonging and Resilience in Individuals with Developmental Disabilities*, Emerging Issues in Family and Individual Resilience, https://doi.org/10.1007/978-3-030-81277-5_6

along with thousands of people, from chaplaincy in institutional settings to community-based ministries, spiritual leaders have been challenged with developing ministries that welcomed and engaged all persons within the worshipping community, regardless of ability. While many well-intentioned spiritual leaders developed segregated ministries *for* individuals with IDD, leaders in the inclusive ministry movement across faiths and theologies focused on developing ministries *by* and *with* individuals with IDD (Gaventa, 2006; Herzog, 2006, 2017). For several decades now, leaders of inclusive faith supports have been thinking about the way inclusion relates to belonging. In the early 1990s, I wrote a short piece for a themed issue on Religion for *The Disability Rag* entitled, "From Believing to Belonging to Believing" (Gaventa, 1993). The premise of the article was that inclusive faith supports should move away from worrying about the capacity for reason by people with intellectual disability and the question of whether or not individuals with intellectual disability could adequately *believe* or *understand* in order to be included. Instead, the focus of inclusive ministries must be on **belonging**, without an intellectual test. But, for belonging to happen, the real question was what professional and laypersons across both faith communities and secular supports and services would **believe** about the importance of belonging, and how committed we would be to put those beliefs in to action. A former institutional chaplain, now working in quality assurance, cut to the heart of our service systems when he commented to me at the 1987 American Association on Mental Retardation, now the American Association on Intellectual and Developmental Disabilities national conference: "We don't really know how to enhance the commitment [of caregiving staff] and so we rely upon compliance" (Gaventa, 2008, p. 599). Shortly after the birth of the Institute on Theology and Disability in 2010 (a 4-day multi-faith institute for theologians, clergy, seminarians, laypersons, faith leaders and others), the 2012 Institute opened up questions about "What's beyond inclusion?" The answer that emerged was belonging (Swinton, 2012).

During the same span in the1980s and 1990s, interdisciplinary research on the relationship between spirituality and health began to explore the impact of spirituality on, among other things, physical health, mental health, recovery, and resilience in the general population. Still, the relationship between spirituality and health in the lives of people with IDD and their families was by and large ignored. There were multiple reasons for this exclusion, including scientific unease with religion in the arena of disability, oral traditions in families and people with IDD about wounding experiences in faith communities, and misunderstandings of the boundaries of church, state, and funding sources (Gaventa, 2018). More recently, focused publications like the "Journal of Disability and Religion" and increasing research published in more scientific journals (e.g. Bertelli et al., 2019; Miller & Skubil-Peplaski, 2020; Narayanasamy et al., 2005) are enhancing current understanding of the interplay between spirituality and IDD.

This chapter begins with a brief exploration of the emerging literature on the interaction of spirituality, belonging, and resilience, followed by the introduction of a conceptualization of spirituality developed from core values that shape services and supports alongside people with IDD and their families. The conceptualization comes out of working with many different faith traditions and within primarily secular systems of service and explores how spirituality across faith traditions implicitly permeates the lives of individuals, families, and service/support systems. Further, this chapter will look at how spirituality can be more explicitly addressed by developing inclusive faith supports. Finally, the goal is to indicate how spirituality can illuminate what can help people participate in faith communities and community life in ways that enhance belonging and resilience among individuals with IDD and their families.

6.1 Defining Terms: Spirituality, Belonging, and Resilience as Constructs of Human Experience

To talk or write about belonging in an inclusive way requires the recognition and incorporation of spirituality. The same is true about the relationships of both belonging and spirituality to the dynamic processes of resilience. The fact that Carter's (this volume, Chap. 2) ten dimensions of belonging emerged from research on spirituality and participation in faith communities among families of individuals with IDD speaks volumes about the importance of spirituality at the heart of meaning-making and the experience of true community. In turn, healthy spirituality, identity, and participation in a supportive faith community are directly tied to solid foundations for individual, family, and community resilience. The same is true about the relationship of both constructs to the dynamic process of resilience. In fact, it is difficult to explore the relationship between any two of these constructs without including the third.

6.1.1 Spirituality

Spirituality, belonging, and resilience are all constructs, a way to define a set of experiences, feelings, behaviors, and thoughts that are not so much empirical and objective as they are relational and subjective. Discerning and naming what is "good, true, valuable, meaningful and decisive in our lives and our parallel worlds belongs to the domain of both religion and science including psychiatry" (Jakovljevic, 2017, p. 238). For researchers in the world of the sciences, defining what is good, true, and beautiful in the world is one of using the objective processes and languages of observing, measuring, and replicating (Gaventa, 2018). However, such reliance upon objective measurements is not the case for the humanities, the arts, and spirituality where languages of identity, community, values, character, and belief are much different, represented and described through their use of story, art, music, symbol, metaphor, and ritual (Gaventa, 2018). The three constructs are also deeply contextual and cultural, with a corresponding expansive diversity of belief and practice.

Spirituality is often defined by its similarities and differences with the word *religion*. Pastoral theologian John Swinton defines spirituality as "the human quest for meaning, purpose, self-transcending knowledge, meaningful relationships, love and absolute value, as well as the sense of the Holy amongst us" (Swinton, 1999, p. 115). Physician and psychiatrist Christina Puchalski, a pioneer in the understandings of spirituality and health, led international efforts to define spirituality as:

> …a dynamic and intrinsic aspect of humanity through which persons seek ultimate meaning, purpose, and transcendence, and experience relationship to self, family, others, community, society, nature, and the significant or sacred. Spirituality is expressed through beliefs, values, traditions, and practices. (Puchalski et al., 2014, p. 646)

Religion, while closely related, "is the expression of the person's spiritual relationship with particular beliefs, practices, rituals that have been developed within a community with others who share a similar understanding and belief system" (Pargament, 1997, p. 27). While one can easily find multiple other similar definitions of both terms, definitions of spirituality often include three key words: meaning, purpose, and connection (to others and to the sacred). Those concepts aligned with the three major dimensions of spirituality that evolved over the course of decades of my work with people with IDD and their families.

"I am *spiritual* but not *religious*" is a common short phrase that covers a depth of personal history and experience and usually indicates some form of disillusionment with or rejection of typical features of organized religion. The power of organized religion or particular religious beliefs to hurt and harm as well as to heal and help is evident in many periods of history, cultures, and dimensions of modern life. This is certainly true in the human experience of IDD, where religious beliefs are used far too easily to diagnose causes (e.g., sin or something someone or their parents did) and/or prescribe cures (e.g., "If you had enough faith, then…"). I use the word "easily" for two reasons. First, people are quick to pass on cultural and colloquial answers to the profound questions raised by IDD, and, second, they have not done the work to understand multiple other ways that IDD has been addressed in religious traditions. The phrase "I am spiritual but not religious" is also a reflection of Western individualism, understandings of freedom, and privacy. One of the root meanings of the word "religion" is that of connections that bind. Thus, while "bind" can seem constrictive, religion also reflects connections and bonds that lead to community and belonging (Gaventa, 2018). The key questions about spirituality center on how it is expressed in community, moves one toward community, and/or helps build meaningful community.

6.1.2 Belonging

Meaningful connections with others and, in both spiritual and religious terms, with a sacred power, are the prime ingredients of belonging. Our individual challenge is often to grow into our sense of personal identity—to answer "Who am I?" The key question of belonging is "Whose am I?" The two questions are closely related, because many of the ways we describe ourselves connect us with others (e.g., nationality, race, religion, roles, politics, skills, occupations, hobbies, sports). Inclusion in the groups and organizations that represent one's shared interests is a key first step. Inclusion enables one to participate. Movements toward inclusion usually focus on rights and places. In contrast, moving toward belonging focuses on relationships and mutuality. We can use the word "belong" to signify possession, but it can also be understood as being in the place where something, or someone, is supposed to be (e.g., my home, my synagogue, my community, my club, my team).

> To belong you need to be missed. People need to be concerned when you are not there; your communities need to feel empty when you are not there. The world needs to be perceived as radically different when you are not there. Only when your absence stimulates feelings of emptiness will you know that you truly belong. Only when your gifts are longed for can community truly be community. (Swinton, 2012, p. 183)

6.1.3 Resilience

A healthy spirituality and the kinds of strong social connections and supports that come from belonging are then frequently cited as two of the key ingredients of resilience. Research from various fields has explored multiple aspects of resilience. Like spirituality and belonging, it too defies objectification. There are multiple definitions such as these insights from rehabilitation and counseling:

> Resilience is considered a multidimensional, dynamic construct made up of a variety of personal qualities (i.e., spirituality, personal competence, social competence, family cohesion, social resources, and personal structure). Individuals who possess these personal qualities are more likely to positively adapt when exposed to a traumatic event…Despite the fact that there is not a single, universal definition of resilience, there are similarities among the qualities believed to characterize resilience, and these include (a) psychological and dispositional attributes, (b) family support and cohesion, and (c) external support systems…Resilience literature also considers spirituality to be a critical source of external support in helping individual's overcome adversity. (White et al., 2008, pp. 9–10)

Another example highlights the role of spirituality in particular:

> Spirituality can enhance resilience by promoting a sense of coherence, hope, transcendental meaning and purpose, and by social support within spiritual community…A fundamental component of the success of any communities is their ability/capacity to collectively build resilience in the face of constant and unpredictable change and adversary. (Jakovljevic, 2017, p. 239)

One important facet noted by both comments is that resilience can be a quality of individuals, families, and communities. All three of the core constructs of spirituality, belonging, and resilience have both individual and communal dimensions that actively influence one another. As noted, personal growth in spirituality leads one into community. A strong sense of personal identity in terms of connections with others gives to and receives from bonds with others. Resilient individuals help build resilient communities, and vice versa. The interdependent dynamism of the three levels of resilience makes them difficult to diagnose into either cause and effect, intervention and impact, or prescription and cure. For that we should be grateful, because otherwise our research and interventions would turn into processes that might assume control.

We have increasingly learned the importance of belonging and resilience in the lives of people with IDD and their families. Paying more attention to the role of spirituality thus makes perfect sense.

6.2 Spirituality and Intellectual and Developmental Disabilities

One of the greatest gifts many professionals have received from our vocational roles in services and supports alongside people with IDD and their families has been the way we have learned from both individuals and families through spiritual insights, core lessons about belonging (or the lack thereof), and their resilience in the face of multiple difficulties. Rather than applying another theoretical understanding of spirituality to IDD, my framework for understanding and describing spirituality evolved out of relationships and learning from relationships with people with IDD, their families, and colleagues within the field of IDD. Understanding spirituality involves addressing the core questions at the heart of five key values built into the policy foundations of disability in the United States and other Western countries: independence, productivity, inclusion, cultural competence, and self-determination (Gaventa, 2018). Table 6.1 highlights how these five values outlined in current policy intersect with common spiritual questions and dimensions of spiritual life, with the final column noting what policies and practices can be used by provider organizations to both address spirituality and enhance belonging (Gaventa, 2018).

Another way to help envision spirituality in the lives of people with IDD and their families is to consider whether spirituality is thought of and supported as a segment of life (see Fig. 6.1) or as the core dimension of our lives as individuals, families, and communities (see Fig. 6.2). Neither is solely correct. Moving our thinking and conceptualizations from a place of *either/or* to *both/and* is in a dimension of the embrace and affirmation of paradoxes in a spiritual perspective. Figure 6.1 can help us think about the ways that families, service systems, and faith community supports can collaborative work together to support individuals with IDD. Figure 6.2 is way of exploring the spiritual dimensions at the heart of individuals and families, faith communities and service systems, and the communities in which we all live.

Going further, there has been an ever-growing body of resources (theological, religious education, family ministries, scriptural, and more) coming out of faith communities in the past 20 years that are accessible as written, video, and personal resources to tap to build inclusive congregations and belonging (see available

Table 6.1 Values, spirituality, and practice

Policy value	Spiritual question	Spiritual themes	Policy/practices
Independence	*Who am I?*	Identity	Person-centered language and planning enhance growth toward independence and interdependence
		Meaning	
Productivity	*Why am I?*	Purpose	Employment
		Calling	Volunteering
		Vocation	Making a difference
		Contribution	
Integration/ inclusion	*Whose am I?*	Community	Community inclusion
		Connection	Community participation
			Least restrictive environment
			Citizenship
			Friendships
Cultural competence	*Where have I come from?*	Traditions	Person-centered planning
	Where are "my people"?	Rituals	Connections
		Worldviews	Honoring choice and uniqueness
Self-determination	*How do I shape my own destiny?*	Choice	Advocacy rights Empowerment
		Control	
		Power	

Note. Adapted from *Disability and spirituality: Recovering wholeness*, p. 71, by W. Gaventa, 2018, Baylor University Press. Adapted with permission

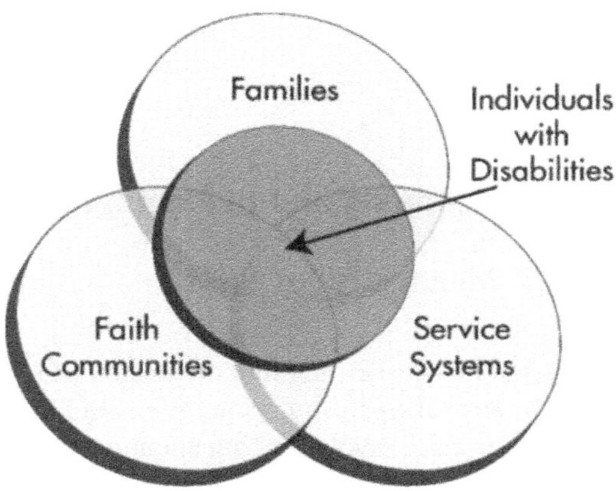

Fig. 6.1 Individual connections to family, service systems, and faith communities

resources from the Collaborative on Faith and Disability, All Belong, Inc., National Catholic Partnership for Disability, and the Ruderman Family Foundation Synagogue Inclusion Project). Many, of course, come out of particular religious traditions, but good resources can be adapted to other kinds of faith communities. For the purpose of this exploration on spirituality and belonging, the discussion will focus on using the five spiritual dimensions in Table 6.1 as well as Figs. 6.1 and 6.2.

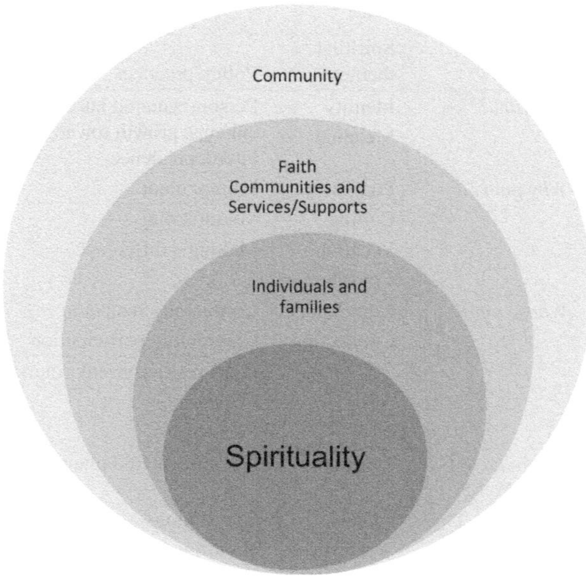

Fig. 6.2 Spirituality at the heart of individuals and communities

The question then becomes: How can we address the spiritual dimensions of the lives of individuals with IDD and their families in ways that build spiritual supports that enhance belonging? Let's start with the spiritual questions of who, why, and whose we are, which include some suggestions of what we can do and how we can do it.

6.3 Spirituality and Belonging: From Theory to Action

6.3.1 Identity: Who Am I?

As mentioned earlier, the first dimension of spirituality revolves around a person's identity, answering the question "Who am I?". The questions "Who am I?" or "Who is someone else" involve asking about one's core values, preferences, and passions; religious and core cultural identities; and what brings meaning to life. A broader question than "What do I believe?", the question of identity aims to decipher what is most central, most sacred to someone's identity (i.e., a person's core values). As offered in the person-centered planning process, *Essential Lifestyle Planning*, the question "What is most important *for* you?" must be balanced with "What is most important *to* you?" (Smull & Sanderson, 2009).

Good person-centered planning realizes one's identity. A simple exercise I have adapted from social psychology (Kanagawa et al., 2001) to help individuals determine their identities only requires a simple sheet of paper. At the top, I write or instruct the individual to write down "I am…" or "[name] is…". Then, I direct them to write at least ten words that are part of their identity. They can use roles, affiliations, hobbies, passions, qualities, or relationships, but not job titles as I find that our work and careers are too often the only identities we think we have. If completed as part of person-centered planning, I often help build the list. If completed in a group, I invite each individual to share their ten words. I often find that individuals write down interests and hobbies, relationships, and key roles, as well as religious identities (e.g., Baptist, Catholic, Jewish) and/or other groups that shape who we are (e.g., Yankee fan, music lover, nature lover). But people very rarely write down or share negative qualities, such as a label of a health condition (e.g., alcoholic) unless in a positive way (e.g., cancer survivor).

Nobody likes being defined through one quality, role, or characteristic, particularly the ones with negative cultural assumptions and connotations. Interestingly, a singular descriptor placed on someone by others and that comes with negative cultural assumptions and connotations is far too often the primary identity for people who have IDD (unless, of course, that individual has learned to take a culturally negative label and turn it into a statement of pride; e.g., "I am black!" or "I am autistic"). Yet, we are all more than one story. Despite common beliefs in the modern world that we are the masters of our story, we are people with many stories, many of which are passed down or given to us, and, in fact, it is the shared stories within our identity that make us interesting to one another. Nigerian writer, Chimamanda Ngozi Adichie (2009), says this brilliantly in her famous TED talk, *The Danger of a Single Story*:

> All of these stories make me who I am. But to insist on only these negative stories is to flatten my experience and to overlook the many other stories that formed me. The single story creates stereotypes, and the problem with stereotypes is not that they are untrue, but that they are incomplete. They make one story become the only story… Power is the ability not just to tell the story of another person, but to make it the definitive story of that person. (Adichie, 2009)

Facilitating more relationships and experiences that lead to multiple stories of identity thus should be a primary jumping off place for both faith communities and agencies committed to enhancing belonging. We must remember that while good person-centered planning processes can foster identity development, it can also be done over cups of coffee, meals together, and shared conversation. The primary tool is story—the primary invitation: "Tell me about yourself." Related specifically to spirituality, the questions and stories may sound like "Do you consider yourself a spiritual or religious person? If so, tell me how and some of your experiences related to that?"—to a parent of a child with IDD, "Tell me about your child?" To ask questions and invite stories is practicing the ancient form of assessment. In today's society, *assessment* often involves a search for a label or diagnosis and includes a process in which a professional stands over and attempts to capture a series of problems or issues. However, the Latin root to the word *assessment* actually means "to sit next to." When we sit next to someone, inviting and listening to their stories, we get to know who they are and the dreams of who they would like to be (Hilsman, 1997).

In terms of spiritual and/or religious identity, think of the way identity is formed while growing up in a faith community. Identity that is formed through official rites of passage and multiple forms of worship, ritual, education, recreation, service, experience, and learning. Think of the stories you heard, or perhaps the experiences you had, of the transforming quality of inclusive rites of passage (Trachtman, 2008). Think of the ways those experiences would help people of all abilities to learn the customs and practices of any faith community, the so-called hidden curriculum, which becomes glaringly apparent when people are included who have no idea or practice how one is supposed to behave in your form of worship or gathering. How do we learn those practices?—by practice, practice, practice, and more practice. Think of the cultural norm then of a person with IDD being able to say: I am_____ . I belong to____ .

Part of our job, whether religious or secular, professional or friendly, is to support people with IDD to have experiences that contribute to more than one story. In turn, we use what we learn about one's story to connect them to people who share similar stories, qualities, interests, or passions. Those parts of identity and spirituality are by no means limited to faith communities.

6.3.2 Purpose: Why Am I?

The answer to the question "Why am I?" all too often is associated with one's employment or line of work. But the deeper question is one focused on purpose: "What do you really like to do?" "Who do you want to be?" "What do most want to do in the world?" Or, in the words of faith traditions, "What is your calling?" "Who are you meant to be?" "What are your gifts?" "What kind of difference would you like to make in the world?"

Starting with passions and interests and moving into experiences and roles where one's interests can be expressed is the starting point to helping people find and fulfill a purpose. Purpose can be lived out through all kinds of roles and relationships A core part of most people's sense of purpose is that they would like to make a difference to others and the world, to give as well as receive. Thus, for service agencies, transition planners, and creative employment programs, it is about giving people the opportunities to test out their interests and passions to find something meaningful to them.

In terms of faith communities, the question beyond inclusion is how do we help people, with and without IDD, find roles within faith communities where they are giving as well as receiving, being disciples as well as being discipled, doing mitzvot, serving as well as being served, and/or giving charity to others.[1] For people with disabilities, the danger of a singular story across history has been that society makes them solely recipients or the consumers. Congregations must fight against this

[1] These expressions of giving as well as receiving represent varied faith communities and traditions.

mental model of disability and stereotype of individuals with disabilities by exploring each person's calling. Find out what someone's interests are, what they might like to do to help out the congregation, and then get them a job that realizes this purpose and calling. There is no faster route to inclusion and belonging in a congregation than for others in a faith community to witness a person with IDD in a role that benefits the life and spirit of the congregation. Usher, greeter, acolyte, setter-upper, taker-downer, nursery or teacher aide, coffee-hour, or shared meal staff—the list goes on and on. If we cannot find a way for a person to use their gifts, even with the support of others, it says more about our lack of creativity than it does about their abilities. If belonging means being missed, visible and valued roles in which people get to know one another is one critical way to help that happen.

There are more steps by which faith communities can assist people with IDD in finding roles meaningful to them. The *Putting Faith to Work* project (Gaventa et al., 2014) is built on a simple premise: faith communities have two amazing forms of social capital. One is their capacity to gather a group around someone in need, especially when that person is known to them. The second is the often overlooked and untapped potential for networking. Social networking is how many people find jobs. You know somebody who knows somebody. Using simple forms of person-centered planning, the premise was that a congregation could gather around an individual with IDD, and, as needed, their family, to get to know the individual, their interests, strengths, and gifts, and what kinds of jobs they might like to try. Then, leveraging the networking power inherent in the whole congregation (full of employees and employers) could be tapped to help someone find a job where they could use their interests, passions, and purpose. For young adults with IDD transitioning out of school and trying to find roles as adults in the community they have grown up in doesn't require a new program, but simply a network that can be tapped into. When that network, such as a congregation, already knows them by name and by their interests, passions, and purpose, it is even better. The *Putting Faith to Work* model is nonsectarian, adaptable to varied contexts and communities, and amendable to collaboration between secular services and faith communities.

6.3.3 *Community and Belonging:* Whose am I?

In all of the major faith traditions, the question of "*Whose* are we?" is more important than "*Who* are we?" That is the major identity question in the *Bible*, *Torah*, and *Qur'an*. A core religious tenet is that everyone is created in the image of God, and part of God's people, however defined. In more secular terms, we sometimes ask "Who are your people?" Answers for many include a combination of ancestry, place, and community belonging, connecting us to (1) time (ancestors), (2) nature, (3) place, (4) people (e.g., family, organizations, communities, colleagues), (5) one self, and (6) the sacred, however defined.

The starting point for thinking about enhancing community and belonging is back at an expanded form of the dimensions of identity identified in response to

"Who am I?" Some parts of our personal and communal identity are given to us at birth, such as culture, ethnicity, race, and gender. (Being given to us does not mean we do not struggle with them, or seek to change them, as we grow.) Others we grow into, such as a faith identity, which are often inherited from our family. Still others emerge from our personal choices, interests, passions, and sense of purpose.

I spent years in my professional roles trying to figure out ways to build and enhance relationships between people with and without IDD, through inclusive worship, recruiting volunteers for respite care programs and other ministries, and learning with others committed to community building through writings and conferences (e.g., Amado, 1993; McKnight, 1995; O'Brien & O'Brien, 1996; O'Connell, 1988; Schwartz, 1997; Vanier, 1989).

Along the way, I finally realized that community building and belonging does not start from deficits (Kretzmann & McKnight, 1993). Relationships and connections are best built on parts of identity other than IDD. Starting with deficits too often leads to services and systems. Gifts and interests lead to connection and community (McKnight, 1995). Figure 6.3 acknowledges that building reciprocal, informal relationships between people with and without IDD in community settings can be difficult. The paradox is that the best path to reciprocal relationships may be indirect. So then, what is the "third thing," the moderating variable, that can bridge the gap between two people and strengthen the connection in their relationship?

Using the interests and passions of a person considered "other" or outside the community, how might we find people in the community with whom interests can be shared? While it is common for persons already in shared community, even temporary shared community based on shared space (e.g., planes, coffee shops), to dive quickly into conversations that explore shared interests and passions, when we view a person from a singular identity of "other," as IDD is often viewed, the gap between persons suddenly appears unbridgeable. We must move from seeing individuals with IDD in our congregations not as other, but as united by shared interests and passions. To get there, we must begin seeing all community members as persons with unique interests and passions and begin making connections based on shared identities, regardless of ability (Gaventa, 2012, 2018).

Carter (2014) shares a powerful story that unfolded when a church in Wisconsin was approached by a nearby group home who had five men with IDD interested in attending the church. In a desire to be welcoming, the pastor made an announcement inviting the congregation to a meeting after the service for anyone interested in being part of a group that would welcome and get to know these men with

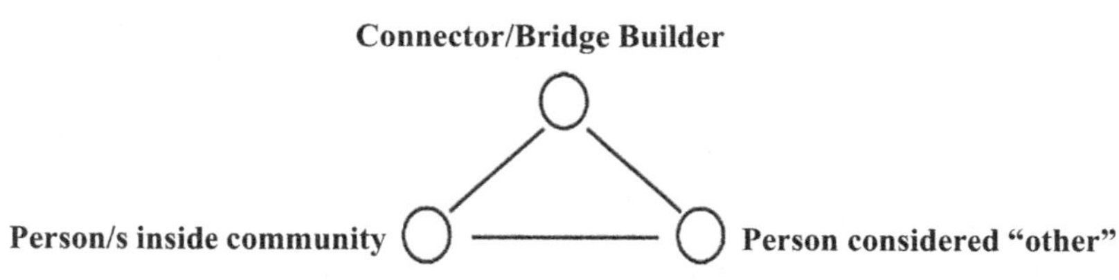

Fig. 6.3 Who, what, and why leads to where, when, and how

IDD. Nobody showed. A couple folks from the church decided to visit the group home and get to know the men. After learning they were huge Green Bay Packers fans, the pastor shared a new and revised announcement to the congregation. He invited all of the men to meeting after church if they were interested in getting together on Sunday afternoons to watch the Packers games. More than 50 men showed up. At the meeting, the men were told there were five Packers fans living in the group home in the neighborhood who never get a chance to watch games with other Packer fans, much less go to a bar or somewhere else and have a beer, or some other socially appropriate habit, like wearing cheese hats. The response of the men from the church was that they thought that was terrible. The leaders then said, "We are going to work on including them in this. We will help you if you have questions about IDD, but you guys know how to be Packer fans." This style of introduction of shared interest switched the focus from the potential fears about IDD or its being a "tragedy" to the tragedy of isolation, and to seeing the lack of opportunity to live out of interests and passions with others as the real problem.

As with all relationships, once started, there is no telling how many other points of connection and shared interests are likely to develop. A key point is that the relationships are thus begun around shared strengths and gifts, not deficits such as "not knowing how to relate to someone with IDD." This same, simple process of relationship development holds true forging the steps that lead to inclusion and belonging of individuals with IDD in faith communities. There are so many potential forms of shared interests and activities in faith communities that the potential for relationships begun on shared passions multiples exponentially.

The questions by the top circle in Fig. 6.3 illustrate ways to help initiate relationships around which communal identity and belonging can be fostered. *What* interests or passions might connect persons both inside and outside of the current community? *Who* shares these interests or passions? *Where do people who share those interests meet?* How might someone get invited and introduced? *When* do they meet? *How* does one become a member or regular participant? What's expected? Who do we know there who could help us?

Interestingly, these questions bring us back around to perhaps the most important question underlying spiritual communal identity—the question of purpose: *Why are we*? While provider agencies' answers to this question focus on goals of community inclusion and other values stated in their mission statements and state policies, local faith communities, churches, and congregations answer that question in ways that vary by their tradition and often within a specific tradition. In broad strokes, one could say that the major faith traditions see their purpose as worshipping and serving God, and, as the "golden rule" states, loving their neighbors as themselves (Rost, 1986). When working with specific congregations and faith communities, community builders and connectors need to understand how that particular community sees itself and its mission. Then, tailored efforts at inclusion and belonging can be developed to meeting their sense of purpose and living out their communal faith as they see it.

6.4 From Theory to Theology and Inclusive Faith Supports

The starting points for connections and relationships outlined above aim to provide a foundation for fostering belonging within both faith communities and secular service and support organizations and networks. While the information presented in Table 6.1 indicate some of the current policies and practices that can be used by service and support organizations to build relationships that have the potential to enhance belonging, more effective methods of community participation and inclusion should be explored, created, and shared. However, as professionals, advocates, and faith community leaders, asking these questions of and to the people we support also requires we ask ourselves the same questions and learn from the ways we have sought out community connections and belonging reflective of our core values and interests (Gaventa, 2018). Funding levels and staff turnover make it very hard for people doing the most direct supports to shoulder the work of building and enhancing relationships. Beginning to think of all of an agency's staff as potential networkers and community builders may be the place from which to start (Gaventa, 2016).

A common consensus has arisen among the leaders of inclusive faith communities that when starting inclusion initiatives within a faith community, involvement of the leadership is crucial. That does not mean that a pastor, rabbi, or imam has to lead the initiatives, but it does mean that they need to support it, bless it, address it in sermons, and help do the connecting that can empower a congregation's work. Faith community leaders can also help articulate how welcoming, including, and supporting people with IDD and their families fits into their congregation's mission and purpose, encourage the congregation to reflect on what is being learned as more inclusive practices develop, and utilize their own faith tradition scriptures and theology to deepen inclusive learning and visioning that fosters belonging. Faith leaders who desire true belonging for all members in their congregation, regardless of abilities, may well find that the language of inclusion and the dimensions of belonging explored in this book are invaluable contributions to the language, symbols, rituals and sacred stories of inclusion and belonging of their particular faith tradition.

Carter's (2016) ten dimensions of belonging as described in Chap. 2 of this book make clear another key principle for practice, namely, that the lessons about what it means to belong for individuals with IDD and their families is really no different than what it means for everyone else. To state it another way, when a question arises about inclusion and belonging related to a person with an IDD in a congregation or any other community setting, the question needs first of all to be reversed and asked about how we would answer the same question for anyone else (Gaventa, 2018). There are countless resources related to best practices for fostering belonging in faith communities and community settings, for example, "Believing, Belonging, Becoming," a short video with four vignettes from different faith communities illustrating stories of inclusion with both children and adults with IDD (Wisconsin Developmental Disabilities Council, 2001), suggesting that the corresponding answers or strategies adapted for enhancing belonging for individuals with IDD will indeed prove mutually beneficial for all community members without disabilities.

Other examples include initiatives to make a congregation accessible for the sake of people who use wheelchairs turn out to help others with less visible support needs (e.g., people who use canes, families who use strollers). A more complex example involves issues of behavior in religious education programs and the "hidden curricula" of attendance and participation. Strategies like positive behavior support training for teachers and helping develop explicit, detailed ways for teaching how to participate most fully in congregational rituals and traditions will benefit other children as well (Gaventa, 2018). Paying attention to inclusive faith supports across the lifespan with families can also bring new life to rituals of transition and membership, such as a bar or bat mitzvah ceremony captured in the beautiful documentary *Praying with Lior* (Trachtman, 2008).

As faith communities learn to include and support all people more effectively, the community not only lives out its faith but also becomes more resilient in responding to new questions and challenges, such as how to be hospitable to the stranger, in whatever form that stranger comes. Seeing every person as possessing unique gifts that can be shared and used in a faith community builds the foundation for supports and participation for everyone, which in turn, becomes a source of resilience for everyone.

6.5 The Greatest of These Is Love

While the focus of community inclusion for people with IDD has too often been location, location, location, the new mantra for belonging moves our focus to relationship, relationship, relationship. It is not enough for individuals with IDD to be *present* in our congregations; we must make efforts to ensure we foster meaningful relationships through which they feel *invited*, *welcomed*, *known*, *accepted*, *supported*, *heard*, *befriended*, *needed*, and *loved* (see Carter, 2016, this volume, Chap. 2). As relationships of belonging are started, honored, preserved, and maintained within faith communities, new and deeper personal and communal dimensions of identity are fostered.

There seems to be some serendipity and providence in triads along the journey toward belonging. Figure 6.3 illustrated the relationships triad, reminding us that relationships between any two persons are often strengthened by a third entity (e.g., interests, passions, places). The model of spirituality described in this chapter also focused on a triad of questions: *Who am I? Why am I?* and *Whose am I?* and the related dimensions of identity/meaning, purpose, and belonging. Those dimensions are woven into one another, in ways that can strengthen the whole, or, if one is very weak, such as persistent and chronic *loneliness*, one's identity and purpose can be negatively impacted as well.

I am taking the liberty now of using a part of my own Christian tradition, but there are parallels in other spiritual and religious traditions. One of the most powerful models of belonging in the New Testament of the *Bible* is described by Paul in his First Letter to the Corinthians, the 12th chapter, that of everyone being part of the "body of Christ." In that body, Paul notes that no one part can claim superiority over another, because every part is needed, every part has a role, and, indeed, some of the "weaker" parts may be much more important than we think. Thus, simply, we all belong.

But Paul does not end there and goes on from an objective metaphor about being connected and bound to one another to what he calls "a more excellent way." No matter what I say or do, he says in essence, "If I have not love, I am nothing." Paul's trinity of values are faith, hope, and love. Translated into the framework of this discussion on spirituality, faith is the equivalent of meaning, what is most important to someone, their core identity. Who are you, all the way down? Hope is then crucial to answering the why question, to seeking and finding purpose, developing resilience to meet challenges and unexpected struggles, and to acting on that sense of vocation and call, being who you were meant to be, finding ways to contribute and make a difference. Finally, love is the force that can power connection and belonging. Each, he seems to say, helps keep the others afloat when one is in trouble, but in the end, love (an acting out of belonging) is the key. We could say this another way, using the languages of public policy and the social sciences, such as "Independence, self-determination, resilience, employment, productivity, and community inclusion are all important, but of them all, community, relationships, and belonging are most crucial to the quality of life of individuals with IDD and their families". But spirituality, belonging, and resilience, as understood and used by everyday people, call for the languages of the humanities and of relationships. Thus, one might say Paul's language is closer to the heart of it all.

Questions for Thought and Discussion

1. Why have service and support systems, as well researchers, been reluctant to address spirituality in the lives of people with intellectual and developmental disabilities and their families?
2. What are the potential benefits and risks in researching the role of spirituality in the lives of people with disabilities and their families as it relates to belonging and resilience?
3. Discuss and share how you respond personally to the core questions of identity, purpose, and belonging.
4. In your envisioned professional role, how might you address and support the spiritual dimensions of the lives of the people whom you serve and support?

References

Adichie, C. N. (2009). *The danger of a single story* [Video]. TED Conferences. https://www.ted.com/talks/chimamanda_adichie_the_danger_of_a_single_story/transcript?language=en.

Amado, A. N. (1993). *Friendships and community connections between people with and without developmental disabilities*. Brookes.

Bertelli, M., Furia, C., Bonadiman, M., Rondini, E., Banks, R., & Lassi, S. (2019). The relationship between spiritual life and quality of life in people with intellectual disability and/or

low-functioning autism spectrum disorders. *Journal of Religion and Health, 59*(4), 1996–2018. https://doi.org/10.1007/s10943-019-00891-x
Carter, E. (2014). *The other six days* [Video]. You Tube. https://www.youtube.com/watch?v=0j51OThheal&feature=youtu.be&t=2191.++Accessed+8%2F18%2F2020.
Carter, E. (2016). A place of belonging: Research at the intersection of faith and disability. *Review and Expositor, 113*(2), 167–180. https://doi.org/10.1177/0034637316637861
Carter, E. W. (this volume). Dimensions of belonging for individuals with intellectual and developmental disabilities. In J. L. Jones & K. L. Gallus (Vol. Eds.), *Belonging and resilience in individuals with intellectual and developmental disabilities – Community and family engagement.* Springer.
Gaventa, W. (1993). From belief to belonging to belief: Trends in ministries with people with mental retardation and their families. *Disability Rag/Resource, 14*(3), 27–29.
Gaventa, W. (2006). Signs of the times: Theological themes in the changing forms of ministries and spiritual supports with people with disabilities. *Disability Studies Quarterly, 26*(4) https://doi.org/10.18061/dsq.v26i4.815
Gaventa, W. (2008). Re-kindling commitment: Reflections from a pastoral educator enmeshed in direct support professional workforce development and person centered supports. *Journal of Intellectual Disability Research, 52*(7), 598–607. https://doi.org/10.1111/j.1365-2788.2008.01070.x
Gaventa, W. (2012). Lessons in community building from including the "other": Caring for one an-other. *Journal of Religion, Disability, and Health, XVI*(4), 231–247. https://doi.org/10.1080/15228967.2012.702415
Gaventa, W. (2016). Presidential address: Re-membering the gifts of professional. *Intellectual and Developmental Disabilities, 54*(6), 454–464. https://doi.org/10.1352/1934-9556-54.6.454
Gaventa, W. (2018). *Disability and spirituality: Recovering wholeness*. Baylor University Press.
Gaventa, W., Allen, W., Kleinert, H., & Carter, E. (2014). *Putting faith to work: The call and opportunity for faith communities to transform the lives of people with disabilities and their communities*. The Vanderbilt Kennedy Center. https://ccids.umaine.edu/wp-content/uploads/sites/26/2015/09/PuttingFaithToWorkPaper91.pdf; http://faithanddisability.org/white_papers/putting-faith-to-work-2/.
Herzog, A. (2006). *Disability history among religious organizations: Histories and reflections*. Routledge.
Herzog, A. (2017). *The social contexts of disability ministry: A primer for pastors, seminarians, and lay leaders*. Cascade Books.
Hilsman, G. (1997). Spiritual pathways: One response to the current standards challenge. *Vision, 7*(6), 8–9.
Jakovljevic, M. (2017). Resilience, psychiatry and religion from public and global mental health perspective dialogue and cooperation in the search for humanistic self, compassionate society and empathic civilization. *Psychiatria Danubina, 29*(3), 238–244. https://doi.org/10.24869/psyd.2017.238
Kanagawa, C., Cross, S. E., & Markus, H. R. (2001). "Who am I?" the cultural psychology of the conceptual self. *Personality and Social Psychology Bulletin, 27*(1), 90–103. https://doi.org/10.1177/0146167201271008
Kretzmann, J., & McKnight, J. (1993). *Building communities from the inside out: A path toward finding and mobilizing a community's assets*. Northwestern University.
McKnight, J. (1995). *The careless society: Community and its counterfeits*. Basic Books.
Miller, V., & Skubil-Peplaski, C. (2020). A systematic review of supports for participation in faith settings for people with disabilities. *Inclusion, 8*(2), 105–123. https://doi.org/10.1352/2326-6988-8.2.105
Narayanasamy, A., Gates, B., & Swinton, J. (2005). Spirituality and learning disabilities: A qualitative study. *British Journal of Nursing, 11*(14), 948–957. https://doi.org/10.12968/bjon.2002.11.14.10467

O'Brien, J., & O'Brien, C. L. (1996). *Members of each other: Building community in company with people with developmental disabilities*. Inclusion Press.

O'Connell, M. (1988). *The gift of hospitality: Opening the doors to community life to people with disabilities*. Northwestern University Center for Urban Affairs and Policy Research. https://www.family-advocacy.com/assets/Uploads/Downloadables/c138365853/10272-The-gift-of-hospitality-Opening-the-doors-of-community-life-to-people-with-disabilities.pdf

Pargament, K. I. (1997). *The psychology of religion and coping*. Guilford Press.

Puchalski, C. M., Vitillo, R., Hull, S. K., & Reller, N. (2014). Improving the spiritual dimension of whole person care: Reaching national and international consensus. *Journal of Palliative Medicine, 17*(6), 642–656. https://doi.org/10.1089/jpm.2014.9427

Rost, H. T. D. (1986). *The golden rule: A universal ethic*. G. Ronald.

Schwartz, D. (1997). *Who cares? Rediscovering community*. Westview Press.

Smull, M., & Sanderson, H. (2009). *Essential lifestyle planning for everyone*. The Learning Community. http://allenshea.com/wp-content/uploads/2017/02/Essential-Lifestyle-Planning-for-Everyone.pdf

Swinton, J. (1999). Reclaiming the soul: A spiritual perspective on forensic nursing. In A. Kettles & D. Robinson (Eds.), *Forensic nursing and the multidisciplinary care of the mentally disordered offender* (pp. 113–127). Kingsley.

Swinton, J. (2012). From inclusion to belonging: A practical theology of community, disability and humanness. *Journal of Religion, Disability & Health, 16*(2), 172–190. https://doi.org/10.1080/15228967.2012.676243

Trachtman, I. (Director). (2008). *Praying with Lior* [Film]. Ruby Pictures.

Vanier, J. (1989). *Community and growth*. Paulist Press.

White, B., Driver, S., & Warren, A. M. (2008). Considering resilience in the rehabilitation of people with traumatic disabilities. *Rehabilitation Psychology, 53*(1), 9–17. https://doi.org/10.1037/0090-5550.53.1.9

Wisconsin Developmental Disabilities Council. (2001). *Believing, belonging, becoming: Stories of faith inclusion* [Video]. YouTube. https://www.youtube.com/watch?v=-9GBNa_5p_k.

Chapter 7
Belonging and Knowledge Production: Fostering Influence Over Science via Participatory Research with People with Developmental Disabilities

Katherine McDonald, Ariel Schwartz, and Micah Fialka-Feldman

Utter the words *developmental disabilities*, and quickly words conveying deficits and images of people without the ability to learn, work, live independently, play, or form relationships with peers and who face early mortality and increased risk for poor health outcomes come to mind. While integrated models of disability (e.g., the social model of disability, the International Classification of Functioning, Disability and Health) are changing how we understand and respond to disability (Kostanjsek, 2011), and thus challenging the inevitability of poor outcomes, we are also learning that some forms of developmental disabilities may offer protection against some health conditions. For example, Down syndrome, a genetically known cause of intellectual disability (and also a developmental disability), appears to promote resilience—or decreased risk—to many forms of cancer (Baek et al., 2009). In the context of these cancers, people with Down syndrome have an advantage over people without the extra chromosome 21.

Identifying the ways individuals with developmental disabilities are resilient, and the ways that socioeconomic factors can further foster resilience, is foundational to promoting the quality of life and human rights for people with developmental disabilities. Importantly, science enables the discoveries that can help us to continuously advance the full inclusion and promote the human rights of all people in society—critical components of authentic belonging (see Carter, this volume, Chap. 2). Yet people with developmental disabilities have a deeply troubled history with science, having long been excluded from respectful engagement with knowledge production. This history has yielded practices that significantly challenge

K. McDonald (✉) · M. Fialka-Feldman
Syracuse University, Syracuse, NY, USA
e-mail: kemcdona@syr.edu

A. Schwartz
Boston University, Boston, MA, USA

J. L. Jones, K. L. Gallus (eds.), *Belonging and Resilience in Individuals with Developmental Disabilities*, Emerging Issues in Family and Individual Resilience, https://doi.org/10.1007/978-3-030-81277-5_7

opportunities to pursue research inclusive of people with developmental disabilities, and thus also thwarts much needed scientific advances. To enhance the ability of new knowledge to promote the quality of life and human rights for all, we must first transform our approach to science. Creating scholarly, scientific environments in which people with developmental disabilities rightly and fully belong is essential to achieving this goal.

7.1 The Far-Reaching Legacy of Past Wrongs: Abuse and Exclusion

The history of science is marred by instances of cruelty and mistreatment of people with developmental disabilities. The earliest recorded transgressions occurred during the Nazi reign in Germany. During this time, people with developmental disabilities were one of the targeted groups subject to abusive treatment under the guise of what was, at the time, framed as medical experimentation. Being subject to these experiments frequently resulted in serious injury and death for people with developmental disabilities (Freedman, 2001). Around the same time, the common practice of placing people with developmental disabilities in large state-run institutions in the United States facilitated easy opportunities for researchers to conduct risky research on individuals widely considered to have little value, often not even perceived as fully human. In these experiments, people with developmental disabilities were harmed, for example, via exposure to viruses or radiation, typically without informed consent and lured to participate by highly coercive incentives such as food or an institutional placement not otherwise available (D'Antonio, 2005; Freedman, 2001).

As these and similar abuses occurring under the guise of science came to light, the public began to speak out and demand accountability and oversight of human experimentation. Informed by international efforts, the National Commission for the Protection of Human Subjects of Biomedical and Behavioral Research (1979) articulated principles to govern the conduct of human experimentation and expanded them to include behavioral research. Today, human experimentation is conducted under greater scrutiny and federal regulations. This system is focused on protective mechanisms designed to prevent abuse and emphasizes key tenets of ethical research, including the importance of voluntary informed consent and offering additional protections when voluntary informed consent is in question, minimizing risks while maximizing benefits, and equitably distributing the risks and rewards of research participation across all members of society (National Commission for the Protection of Human Subjects of Biomedical and Behavioral Research, 1979).

An unintended negative consequence of this protective emphasis has been widespread exclusion from direct research participation and removal of self-determination in research participation decision-making among people with developmental disabilities (Feldman et al., 2014; Jacobson et al., 2013). Researchers may encounter challenges with voluntary informed consent for many people with developmental disabilities because of cognitive impairments, communication barriers, and complex social dynamics. These concerns prompted many institutions to enact policies addressing the inclusion of people with "cognitive impairments" or "questionable capacity to consent" (National Institutes of Health, 2009). While the intent was to protect people from further harm, the result has been widespread exclusion of people with developmental disabilities from research participation, others consenting to research participation on their behalf, and requirements that they demonstrate capacity to understand research procedures and their rights as participants (Dalton & McVilly, 2004; Iacono, 2006; McDonald & Kidney, 2012).

These outcomes have far-reaching consequences. Particularly concerning, systematic exclusion from research participation has meant we know little about people with developmental disabilities and how to promote their full inclusion in all aspects of society, health, well-being, and rights. In many cases, knowledge gained from proxy report (representatives responding about or on behalf of individuals with developmental disabilities) has limited scientific validity and is ethically problematic (McDonald & Raymaker, 2013; Spong & Bianchi, 2018). Widespread exclusion from research participation also reinforces perceptions that people with developmental disabilities are incompetent to participate and unable to contribute to science, conveying the message "you do not belong." In some cases, researchers try to promote inclusion of people deemed unable to consent for themselves by allowing others to consent on their behalf. However, this can lead to people with developmental disabilities being forced unwillingly to participate in research and face risks they might not choose for themselves, or being excluded when they might choose to participate if given the opportunity to decide. Finally, the requirement that people with disabilities must demonstrate capacity to consent constitutes disability-based discrimination and can exclude people with developmental disabilities from pursuing opportunities of personal interest (McDonald & Kidney, 2012; McDonald & Raymaker, 2013; Northway, 2014; Northway et al., 2014).

7.2 Charting a Path Toward Belonging: Inclusion and Influence in Science

Today, we are in the early waves of a transformation. As we increasingly recognize the full rights of people with developmental disabilities to be presumed competent and assert control over their lives, there is awareness that part of securing health equity and full citizenship entails people with developmental disabilities having opportunities to participate directly in research (Spong & Bianchi, 2018). As researchers are called to include people with developmental disabilities as research respondents, researchers are asked to move from proxy consent to first-person consent or meaningful assent and to establish research practices that reflect what people with developmental disabilities perceive as the risks, rewards, and appropriate safeguards (Lory, 2019; McDonald et al., 2013, 2016a, b; McDonald, 2012; McDonald & Raymaker, 2013).

While better inclusion of people with developmental disabilities in research as respondents addresses some errors of the past and fosters important advances in new knowledge to inform full inclusion and equity, it leaves other pressing concerns unresolved. Important concerns unanswered include whose interests are served by prevailing research agendas? Who stands to benefit or be harmed by particular research projects? As we re-examine who has leadership in science and its far-reaching, long-lasting consequences, we are asking new questions such as does the way we distribute research funding match the priorities of people with developmental disabilities? Do research agendas reflect deficit-based frameworks or a human rights approach that considers environmental supports and factors? Do research agendas seek to unearth protective factors that can help individuals fully belong and flourish?

Current answers to these questions are disappointing and fall short of our goals for disability justice. For example, using information from a federal committee, we can examine how modern science addresses these questions in the context of research focused on autism (a developmental disability). After categorizing research funding into seven areas, the Interagency Autism Coordinating Committee (IACC) found that funding allocations favor questions about biological causes, risk factors, and treatments and interventions that seek to "normalize" behaviors (IACC, 2017; Office of Autism Research Coordination et al., 2019). Yet the autistic[1] community is speaking out against such investments, suggesting such funding allocations can yield efforts to eradicate autistic people, promote dehumanizing and maladaptive behaviors such as insistence upon direct eye contact or distinguishing of stimming behaviors (e.g., flapping) that may in the long-term create greater harm than benefit, and deter funding topics of greater value to autistic people (e.g., topics spanning the lifespan and services) (Jaswal & Akhtar, 2018; McDonald & Raymaker, 2013; Nicolaidis, 2012; Nicolaidis et al., 2011).

The IACC findings as well as concerns raised by the autistic community demonstrate how focusing solely on enhancing the inclusion of people with developmental disabilities as research respondents falls short of addressing the systemic discrimination of people with developmental disabilities within science, and the far-reaching implications of this exclusion on whose interests are served and what harms might consequently persist. As we tackle new questions about ethical approaches to science, relying on disability rights suggests how to proceed. The disability rights mantra "nothing about us, without us" (Charlton, 1998) emphasizes full inclusion as a critical strategy for addressing complex ethical questions. As a hallmark of true belonging, this mantra insists that we move beyond inclusion of people with developmental disabilities in science as research respondents to *influence* of people with developmental disabilities over science writ large.

---

[1] For more information on identity-first language, see AASPIRE's use of "person first language." https://aaspire.org/about/aaspires-use-of-person-first-language/.

One way to promote influence over science is to pursue authentic research partnerships with people with developmental disabilities. The success of these efforts resides largely in transforming relationships. More specifically, the relationships of people with developmental disabilities to the system of knowledge production and the actors therein. Partnering with people with developmental disabilities as co-researchers throughout all phases of research, using approaches such as community-based participatory research (CBPR) or participatory action research (PAR), can transform the scientific and ethical merits of research (McDonald & Stack, 2016). Via these partnerships, researchers are able to draw upon the preferences of people with developmental disabilities to determine or refine research questions and identify research procedures that promote first-person consent and meaningful assent, reduce risks, and include protections that foster self-determination and dignity (McDonald & Raymaker, 2013; Nicolaidis et al., 2011). In addition to pursuing participatory research, we need to go further to fully promote influence over science: We also need to pursue the full representation of people with developmental disabilities in agencies and on boards that make research funding decisions and oversee ethical research practices (e.g., Institutional Review Boards [IRBs]), in peer review processes, and as trained scientists leading scientific investigations and educating the next generation of researchers. As a result of these synergistic efforts, we will come to better understand resilience and the environmental protective factors that help people with developmental disabilities lead fulfilling lives replete with the same access to opportunities and outcomes as people without disabilities.

To change the relationships of people with developmental disabilities to the system of knowledge production and the actors therein and to authentically and fully say "you belong," we must change practice as usual. We therefore call upon many individuals and organizations to learn new ways of conducting research and to speak up for what is right. Thanks to pioneering work by teams around the world, we are building our knowledge base of effective ways to promote inclusion in and influence over science so that the message clearly becomes "you belong." At the heart of this work is relationship, and we thus focus here on how researchers can foster belonging in science via transformative relationships.

7.3 Fostering Belonging in Science Through Transformative Relationships

The first step toward fostering belonging in science is to acknowledge that science is inherently relational. As described, historically, relationships between scientists (we use this term hereafter to refer to those with formal academic training in research) without disabilities and people with developmental disabilities have been plagued by ableism, paternalism, and abuse of power (Bottema-Beutel et al., 2020; McDonald et al., 2020). To foster belonging, scientists without disabilities must take responsibility for cultivating more positive relationships and earning the trust of people with developmental disabilities. Below, we describe four areas that emerge from our experience and review of the literature as critical for relationships that transform the current scientific approach and provide the conditions for authentic partnerships. These areas include becoming an ally and advocate for the full inclusion of people with developmental disabilities in science; establishing mutual, long-term relationships with people with developmental disabilities in science; creating structures that show respect and foster engagement, participation, and shared decision-making; and engaging in reflexive practice. As we consider transformational relationships, we focus on the actions scientists without developmental disabilities can take to foster greater belonging of people with developmental disabilities in science.

7.3.1 Become an Ally and Advocate for the Full Inclusion of People with Developmental Disabilities in Science

Many readers likely believe that collaborating with people with developmental disabilities is a good thing to do and that creating more and higher-quality space for people with developmental disabilities in science is needed. While this mindset is an important starting point, it is equally critical for scientists without disabilities to develop a strong foundation in disability history, oppression, and disability rights to avoid perpetuating past injustices and tokenism (or acts that unconsciously reflect ableism), and instead advance disability justice within science. The pervasiveness of deficit-based thinking often leads to implicit bias about the abilities of people with developmental disabilities. Consequently, if scientists without disabilities do not make efforts to directly challenge cultural messages and professional models, they may unconsciously underestimate the potential of people with developmental disabilities to contribute to sciences (e.g., understand the scientific process, provide ideas about how to effectively recruit, interpret the implications or meaning of findings).

Researchers without disabilities can begin educating themselves by reading about disability history, disability rights, and disability studies (e.g., Charlton, 1998; Davis, 2013; Oliver, 1990), watching documentaries (e.g., Habib, 2018; Neudel, 2011), and attending disability culture and recreational events (e.g., performances, demonstrations, museums or museum expositions, inclusive sports expos or games). However, the best education scientists without developmental disabilities can receive is that which comes directly from people with disabilities. As an added bonus, seeking out such relationships allows scientists without developmental disabilities to initiate transformative relationships to enable belonging. Forming relationships with people with disabilities in one's community or by volunteering with self-advocacy groups provides opportunities to understand the day-to-day impact of ableism and exclusion. Importantly, scientists without disabilities can earn the status of "ally" by advocating alongside people with disabilities for their self-described needs, both in the context of civil rights and science. This means not only partnering with people with disabilities in one's own research but encouraging others and working within academic systems to reduce barriers to partnerships with people with developmental disabilities. For example, to fully embody disability rights in science, when scientists are invited to present or to serve on an important decision-making body, such as a grant review panel or IRB, they can invite a person with a developmental disability (or a group of people) to co-present or co-serve and ensure that those invited receive appropriate payment for their professional contributions. Ultimately this may also result in long-term employment at a university for an individual with a developmental disability. One of us (MFF) benefited from university faculty noting his expertise and value and paving the way for long-term employment at the university.

7.3.2 *Establish Mutual, Long-Term Relationships with People with Developmental Disabilities in Science*

Given that that scientific inquiry is inherently relational, it is important to identify strategies for establishing and fostering mutually rewarding, long-term relationships with people with developmental disabilities effective in and appropriate to the context of science. Critical dimensions of these relationships include the selection of community researchers with disabilities, creating community among all research team members, establishing and demonstrating trustworthiness, communication, and transparency about the extent of power sharing or collaboration.

7.3.2.1 Selection of Community Researchers

Critical to beginning successful partnerships is the identification of suitable team members. Research—a sometimes lengthy and tedious process—may not be of interest to all people with developmental disabilities. It is also important to identify team members with shared values, relevant life experiences, and the ability to commit to the time required to complete the research (Embregts et al., 2018; McDonald & Stack, 2016; Nicolaidis et al., 2020; Schwartz et al., 2020a; Strnadova et al., 2016). Community researchers with developmental disabilities who do not have formal academic training in research, but who contribute their lived experience and expertise to research teams, can be recruited through existing relationships and networks, partnering with self-advocacy groups and/or disability services/agencies and job postings. Selection of community researchers with developmental disabilities may be driven by prior knowledge of their interests and skills, in tandem with discussions of their interests in the new partnership and/or formal job interviews. Importantly, when conducting job interviews, they must be made accessible to individuals with developmental disabilities (e.g., provide interview questions ahead of time, communicate using the candidate's preferred mode of communication, etc.) (Schwartz & Durkin, 2020). It is important that all research team members agree upon expectations for collaboration and that these expectations are clearly documented (Nicolaidis et al., 2019; McDonald & Stack, 2016). In one of our community-engaged projects, two of us (KM and MFF) created a document that explained expectations for the project. The document, which was reviewed in multiple formats (print and oral), detailed the roles, responsibilities, and rights of each project member so that everyone understood what they were agreeing to and what they would receive as a result (e.g., compensation, professional opportunities, etc.). Carefully selecting research team members without disabilities—scientific and nonscientific—can also contribute to the success of a partnership. Team members without disabilities must share values of inclusion and disability rights, have strong interpersonal skills, be open to learning from all team members and willing to have flexible work hours, and defer to the preferences of others (e.g., use a less-preferred mode of communication) to accommodate the needs and schedules of team members with disabilities (Garcia-Iriarte et al., 2014; McDonald & Stack, 2016; Schwartz et al., 2020a).

7.3.2.2 Creating Community Among All Research Team Members

Once formed, it is critical to foster a sense of community and belonging among all team members (Bewley & McCulloch, 2006; McDonald & Stack, 2016), which creates the beginning of a partnership. Tools such as creating an accessible video to introduce each team member (e.g., name, photograph, and key personal and professional information they wish to share) and accessible icebreaker activities can facilitate the beginning of relationships. Genuine care for team members can also be demonstrated by regularly including "check-ins" about team members' lives in routine work meetings or less formal personal conversation outside of meetings (traveling together, whether in the context of local transportation to events or meetings or out of town travel, can greatly deepen personal relationships). While prolonged relationships can help foster community and belonging over time (Knox et al., 2000; Schwartz et al., 2020a), coming together for non-research-related activities, such as shared meals or meeting for coffee, and social outings to local events of interest such as Americans with Disabilities (ADA) parades, baseball games, or movies can accelerate and strengthen authentic relationships (The Learning Difficulties Research Team, 2006). Over time, stronger relationships and trust translate into more effective teamwork.

7.3.3 Establishing and Demonstrating Trustworthiness

Trust is a critical component of research partnerships given the bleak history of disability research and ongoing oppression experienced by people with disabilities and must be earned and continuously maintained by scientists without disabilities

(Nind & Vinha, 2012). Trust can also be fostered through transparency in decision-making, consistent follow-through, and clear, flexible, and ongoing communication. Shared decision-making may be achieved via formalized strategies, such as the "five finger method" used by the Academic Autism Spectrum Partnership in Research and Education (AASPIRE) (Nicolaidis et al., 2011, 2019) or voting (Northway et al., 2014).

While ideally all members of the team would be involved in all decisions, doing so isn't always practical or desirable. Nonetheless, scientists should seek to maximize shared decision-making and be transparent about any constraints on shared decision-making. When shared decision-making is not possible, scientists should communicate with team members and provide the rationale behind decisions made without all team members.

Importantly, when community researchers with disabilities express a preference or decision, academic researchers without disabilities must act upon these preferences. Following through on these decisions demonstrates the value of their contributions and knowledge, further fostering belonging (McDonald & Stack, 2016). For example, during the development of a self-advocacy intervention for young adults with developmental disabilities, community researchers with disabilities requested a module about the impact of environmental modifications on others. In their experiences, they preferred advocating for modifications that positively or neutrally impacted others, as opposed to modifications that they felt may make activities less fun or harder for other people involved. While the principal investigator initially had felt it was important to prioritize modifications that would maximize participation, she decided to honor the input and lived experience of the community researchers with disabilities by including this module, which ultimately strengthened the intervention (Kramer et al., 2013). In another one of our projects (MFF, KM), when community researchers with disabilities indicated they preferred working in-person as a group and did not want to communicate via team management software, the academic researchers made these changes to the research team procedures.

Clear, flexible, and ongoing communication can also foster trust. Research teams should conduct meetings in a format that supports all members' communication preferences. For example, after realizing that teleconference meetings were inaccessible for autistic team members, AASPIRE transitioned to conducting meetings using text-based internet chat (Nicolaidis et al., 2011). In contrast, per team member preference, Project ETHICS members worked in person so that everyone could understand information and participate in idea generation, discussions, and decision-making. Project ETHICS team members also preferred frequently using a "round robin" approach, going around the room giving each person an opportunity to address the group on the topic under discussion (McDonald et al., 2016a). Additional approaches to ensure clear communication include use of pictures, plain language, and opportunities for individual thinking, rather than relying on group discussion as a primary means of communication. Teams must be ready to adapt their communication style as new team members join and/or as members' needs change, particularly when individual needs change as team members learn and grow or when project needs change over time (Stack & McDonald, 2018).

Finally, communication must be ongoing to maintain relationships and keep all team members engaged between meetings, and especially phases of the research that require less active engagement of community researchers with developmental disabilities. Some teams may choose to have regularly occurring, in-person meetings to maintain their connections to team members and the project. During less "active" periods of research, these meetings may be primarily to provide updates, such as the timeline for a grant being reviewed, a manuscript being published, or project findings being used to inform a new bill. Communicating about non-research-related events, such as birthdays; a new position or an award for a team member; or resources and events that might be of interest to team members can also help maintain connections.

7.3.4 Be Transparent About the Continuum of Power-Sharing in Research Partnerships and Take Actions that Reflect the Selected Participatory Approach

While disability justice requires people with developmental disabilities be involved in all research about them, the nature and extent of involvement varies, depending on the project and available resources. Given this variability, scientists must be transparent about the nature and extent of involvement of community researchers with developmental disabilities. The extent to which people with developmental disabilities are involved in research ranges from having advisory roles to having equal roles to academic researchers without disabilities to having leading roles. Teams should reserve the terms *community-based participatory research* or *participatory action research*[2] for projects in which academic and community researchers share power and researchers with disabilities are authentically engaged throughout all phases of the research project, from the identification of research questions through dissemination and any actions for knowledge translation or change (Nicolaidis et al., 2019; Stack & McDonald, 2014). Transparency about the type of partnership and the extent of power sharing is critical for fostering and maintaining trust of both disability and research communities; promises of greater power sharing than is actualized is disingenuous and contributes to mistrust.

Participatory research may not be appropriate for all research projects. When scientists ask questions that are not driven by the self-described preferences of people with disabilities, but may benefit from their input, they may opt for less involvement of community researchers with disabilities. For example, a biologist who has discovered that an existing pharmaceutical has a secondary effect of reducing

[2] Approaches to research characterized by equitable, respectful relationships between scientists and community members throughout all phases of research from conceptualization to dissemination and action. Community-based participatory and participatory action research build from community strengths and resources, emphasize co-learning, and combine knowledge and action to promote social justice, health, and well-being.

spasticity may have a fundamental scientific question (e.g., the biological mechanism of action) but also want to explore the acceptability of side effects, whether the use of the pharmaceutical results in outcomes meaningful for people with disabilities, or how to best foster uptake of this new treatment approach. This scientist may recruit an advisory board that provides feedback on outcome measures and dissemination strategies to ensure that potential consumers with disabilities understand the risks and benefits of the pharmaceutical. While the input of the advisory board is invaluable, a participatory approach is not necessarily needed to answer the scientist's primary scientific question, and use of an advisory board alone does *not* constitute participatory research (Seekins & White, 2012). However, the role of the advisory board remains valuable and a worthy endeavor. In other cases, scientists without disabilities may have an established protocol, but realize while preparing their study that the voice of people with disabilities is missing. They may subsequently recruit community researchers with developmental disabilities to be members of their research team and be actively involved in specific components of their project, including refining methods, analyzing and interpreting data, and dissemination. Yet, since the research question and design, and thus, the majority of power reside with the scientists without disabilities, it would not be appropriate to describe the team's approach as participatory. Rather, the team may say they used an "inclusive research" or "collaborative research" approach. Perhaps this team can work together to identify subsequent research questions together, and thus develop a follow-up study that is truly participatory (Bigby et al., 2014; Walmsley, 2004).

Resources may also play a role in decisions about the nature of partnerships and extent of opportunities to collaborate. Participatory approaches are time- and resource-intensive (Stack & McDonald, 2014; Walmsley et al., 2018). All phases of research take longer when working as a team, and community researchers with developmental disabilities may only work a few days each month unless research is their full-time or primary job. Furthermore, additional resources are needed to develop accessible materials and provide additional supports described below (e.g., previewing materials, transportation). Subsequently, there may be times that scientists without disabilities desire to involve community researchers with disabilities throughout the entire research process (e.g., identifying the research question, collecting and analyzing data, dissemination), yet are not able to achieve full power sharing across all phases of research due to lack of time and resources. For example, when developing a peer mentoring intervention for young adults with developmental disabilities and mental health conditions, one of us (AS) partnered with a team of young adults with disabilities. Due to the constraints of the grant, this ten-session program needed to be developed and piloted within 18 months. As a result of community researchers' school and work responsibilities, in addition to budget concerns, the full team only met for 2 hours each week; consequently, the academic researcher (AS) was not able to gather input on all materials for all ten intervention sessions. However, when she developed materials independently, she strove to incorporate previous feedback team members had provided on other, similar materials. While time can limit opportunities for full collaboration, creative solutions can be implemented to nonetheless foster input.

While scientists concerned about power in research may be eager to use a participatory approach across all of their work, it is important to use reflexive practice and honestly examine and subsequently describe the nature of one's work. Transformative relationships and ethical science can exist along the entire range of the continuum of research partnerships. One approach to fostering participatory research partnerships is to cultivate long-term relationships with researches with disabilities by establishing a team that works across multiple projects. Some examples include the Inclusive Research Network in Ireland (Inclusive Research Network, n.d.; Salmon et al., 2018) and AASPIRE in the United States (Nicolaidis et al., 2019). These teams formed in response to a desire to conduct participatory research honoring the rights and self-described needs of people with disabilities, rather than to conduct a specific project. They established protocols for working together and have existed for over a decade, conducting diverse projects, with the research questions, methodology, and dissemination strategies collaboratively chosen. The longevity of these teams facilitates their participatory work, because team members have strong and trusting relationships, established protocols, and capacities built through mutual learning over time (Kidd et al., 2018).

It is important to carry partnerships through to the end of research projects, ensuring community researchers with developmental disabilities are involved in dissemination and subsequent action (e.g., providing information to policy makers or writing a grant for an intervention based on findings from the initial project). This can be challenging if community scientists without disabilities find themselves working on dissemination after formal funding has ended. Yet, it is important for researchers with disabilities to shape dissemination and action approaches to ensure they are meaningful to people with disabilities. Sometimes alternative funding sources, such as discretionary funds that can be allocated by the principal investigator, or university, can support continued engagement in dissemination. Community researchers with disabilities may share findings using a range of approaches, including writing accessible reports, presenting at self-advocacy conferences, creating video reports, and producing photo exhibits (Haigh et al., 2013; O'Brien et al., 2014; Stack & McDonald, 2014). While these outputs may not directly benefit academic researchers without disabilities as much as traditional scientific outputs (e.g., journal articles), they are critical for power sharing and to fully realize the benefits of research for disability communities (Zarb, 1992). Some community researchers with disabilities may want to become involved in writing manuscripts for academic journals. This can take a variety of forms, ranging from reviewing the article and providing feedback to co-writing using accessible strategies such as talking aloud while one person types (Strnadová & Walmsley, 2018). When community researchers with developmental disabilities contribute to manuscript production, which includes review and feedback, their contributions should be acknowledged with authorship.

In many cases, simply reporting research findings may not be adequate for teams who share a vision of directly using research findings to improve the lives of people with developmental disabilities. That is, knowledge translation requires a proactive process beyond academic publications (Straus et al., 2009). Action steps can include using research findings to advocate for changes in services and legislation. When research results in tools and resources, action involves continued efforts for implementation on the ground. Research teams need to ensure that there is sufficient funding to engage in action and support the ongoing engagement of researchers without disabilities in dissemination and action (Stack & McDonald, 2014).

7.3.5 Create Structures that Show Respect and Foster Engagement, Participation, and Shared Decision-Making

It is critical that research teams create an environment that demonstrates respect for the time and expertise of community researchers with disabilities, meets accessibility needs, and privileges the voices of community researchers with developmental disabilities. Importantly, community researchers with developmental disabilities should be compensated for their work. Our research teams, and others, have worked with universities to employ team members with disabilities and provide competitive and appropriate wages, even when our university guidelines for wages based largely on educational attainment provided initial challenges to this goal (Kidney & McDonald, 2014; Schwartz & Durkin, 2020). When this is not possible, team members may be compensated with gift cards or cash, subawards to self-advocacy groups, or payment for work travel such as presentations. Further, because transportation can pose a barrier to engagement, transportation or transportation costs should also be provided (ideally upfront as needing to wait for reimbursement for those living with limited economic means can be difficult or impossible). Providing financial compensation and supporting partners' transportation demonstrates respect for their time, skills, and knowledge and helps assure that community researchers with developmental disabilities receive direct financial benefits from their labor, similar to scientists without disabilities (Frankena et al., 2019; Nicolaidis et al., 2015; Northway et al., 2014). In some cases, researchers with developmental disabilities may express concerns about their salary resulting in the cessation of government benefits, due to benefit eligibility regulations. Scientists without disabilities should address the impact of a salary on benefit eligibility with all team members and work with team members to engage their case managers in the discussion, to ensure there are no unintended consequences of engagement in research or receiving a salary. When receiving a salary for research may lead to disqualification for benefits, team members should work together to agree upon a fair alternative for compensation.

7.3.5.1 Establish Guidelines

Another way to demonstrate respect for team members with developmental disabilities is to collaboratively establish guidelines for how to work together. Doing so can help establish mutually agreeable structures and processes for power sharing at the onset. Two of us (KM and MFF) did this for our projects. In this example, KM proposed a draft set of guidelines created in prior collaborations with people with developmental disabilities to MFF and another community researcher with a developmental disability. After making small refinements, we brought the proposed guidelines to the expert panel (as the participatory group was called in this project). We discussed them as a group, made adjustments based on the group's preferences and needs, and voted to accept them. The guidelines delineated how we showed mutual respect, provided accommodations, and engaged in shared decision-making. We posted the guidelines on the wall of our meeting room and identified a rotating member as the "process monitor" to note if we were departing from these guidelines (McDonald et al., 2016a).

7.3.5.2 Working with Diverse Stakeholders

Guidelines for working together may be particularly important on research teams with diverse stakeholders. For example, some research teams may include community researchers with disabilities, family members, and additional community members, such as doctors, direct support providers, and policy makers. Due to implicit bias, diverse stakeholders, without a deep background in disability history and rights, may be skeptical about the role and involvement of community researchers with disabilities. Group guidelines can ensure that all team members are respected, research activities remain accessible, and high expectations for all team members are upheld.

Collaborative research should be approached with the assumption that community researchers with developmental disabilities have the capacity to engage in the entire process. This capacity can be realized through the use of individualized accommodations (Stack & McDonald, 2014). Below, we discuss many of these accommodations, but note that community researchers with developmental disabilities are the experts on the supports they need. While scientists without disabilities should anticipate the need for accommodations (and budget the resources for them), the first step should be asking community researchers with developmental disabilities for their input on how to make research accessible for them.

To foster engagement and shared decision-making, all research activities and discussions should use plain language (e.g., short sentences, concrete references, avoid research "jargon") and team members' preferred communication approach. Additionally, use of visuals and graphic devices (e.g., flow charts), ensuring materials are compatible with screen readers, and a slower conversation pace can be helpful for many researchers, with and without disabilities (McDonald & Stack, 2016; Nicolaidis et al., 2015; O'Brien et al., 2014). We refer readers to universal design principles (see Nelson, this volume, Chap. 4) as a starting point for thinking about accommodations that may support researchers with heterogeneous strengths and support needs. One-on-one support can also bolster access. Research assistants and other support staff can help community researchers with developmental disabilities throughout the research process by orienting them to materials and agenda items, adapting materials in real-time, and providing immediate clarifications, as needed. Some community researchers emphasize the usefulness of having a "point" person, who they can contact about questions related to research, before, during, and after meetings. In our experience, it can also be helpful to meet with community researchers with developmental disabilities before meetings to preview materials and concepts (Kramer et al., 2019; McDonald et al., 2016a; McDonald & Stack, 2016).

Reducing the cognitive load of research tasks can also increase accessibility. Cognitive load refers to how working memory and executive functioning demands (i.e., "cognitive load") increase when tasks require simultaneous processing of multiple elements or pieces of information (Clark et al., 2011). Cognitive load can be decreased by breaking concepts and tasks into smaller parts. We found actively working to reduce cognitive load particularly useful during qualitative data analysis and interpretation, and other research tasks that are lengthy and abstract. In our approach, we combined the strategy of "breaking down tasks" with universal design approaches to make this complex process as accessible as possible (Kramer et al., 2011; Kramer & Schwartz, 2018; McDonald et al., 2016a; Schwartz et al., 2020b, c). In this approach, scientists without disabilities present each sentence from a verbatim transcript separately and work with community researchers with developmental disabilities to identify the main idea in each sentence. Then, team members sort these main ideas into similar color-coded categories. Next, the team or small groups consider the main ideas in each category to identify overarching "big ideas" (i.e., "themes"). In some cases, team members may move main ideas from one category to another, identify overlap between categories, and/or count how many main ideas are within each category. To summarize the data, team members take turns presenting the "final" main ideas from each category. To scaffold this process, team members may record the presented ideas on a worksheet or large poster, so all "final main ideas" can be seen side by side (Schwartz et al., 2020b, c).

Sometimes, team members have accommodation needs that appear conflicting at first glance. For example, some team members may prefer to communicate via writing or reading, but others may have difficulty reading and writing. Some team members may require technology that speaks to them, while others are sensitive to unexpected or unknown noises in their environments. Some team members may need very short sentences to understand, while others require very precise (and longer) sentences to understand. When conflicting accommodation needs arise, team members can work together to reach a compromise. For example, meetings could be conducted with the simultaneous assistance of communication access real-time transcription (CART), text-to-speech software, and computers, so researchers with auditory processing challenges and researchers with difficulty reading and writing can communicate with each other (i.e., some people can write/read, and others can talk/listen). Finally, as work progresses, team members may find that they need different supports or that the processes for working together change as the nature of the work changes (Stack & McDonald, 2018). Therefore, it is critical to continually reassess the effectiveness of the teams' structures and individualized accommodations to ensure that the team adapts over time as needed or desired for a successful collaboration.

7.3.5.3 Accessing the Lived Experience

Community researchers with developmental disabilities contribute significant expertise based on their lived experiences. It is imperative that researchers' lived experiences are incorporated when developing research questions and data collection approaches, analyzing and interpreting data, and disseminating findings. This expertise can best be incorporated when researchers with disabilities are supported to reflect upon their previous experiences and their implications for the research project. For example, when developing a mental health intervention, a scientist without disabilities (AS) developed worksheets and interactive activities to promote reflection on team members' own experiences with mental health symptoms and treatment. Community researchers with developmental disabilities could then more readily call upon these prior experiences to inform the research. In some cases, it may be difficult to recall or describe past experiences, due to memory and communication demands of recall. Interviews in which researchers with disabilities physically lead another team member through their neighborhood or day (i.e., "go-along interviews"), use of research "diaries," and video/photography can also support partners to reflect on personal experiences relevant to the research topic (Milner & Frawley, 2018; Morgan et al., 2015). When developing a youth self-report measure of daily activities, one team asked community researchers with developmental disabilities to identify meaningful daily activities with varied levels of difficulty (Kramer & Schwartz, 2018). Together, the community researcher with a developmental disability and a scientist without disabilities performed these activities and identified each step of the activity by taking pictures and videos and completing a structured worksheet. This experiential activity promoted reflection and subsequently led to the generation of new content for the self-report measure the team was developing.

7.3.6 Reflective Practice: Learning and Improving Over Time

As noted, team members' needs, team dynamics, and the nature of the work change over time. Therefore, it is important to continually reflect on the relationships, structures, and processes of the team. Some research teams conduct a "check-out" at the end of each meeting to determine what went well and what should be changed to ensure successful and accessible partnerships (McDonald & Stack, 2016; Stack & McDonald, 2018). Other teams have used tools to identify "who did what" at the conclusion of each research activity to support all team members to reflect on their roles in carrying out research activities and decision-making (Garcia-Iriarte et al., 2009). This process also allows everyone to recognize individual contributions and assess whether they are contributing as desired. For example, after working together for 5 years to develop a youth self-report of daily activities, one of our teams (AS) developed "officer" positions to facilitate greater ownership over the research product and ensure ongoing input, even when the full team was not able to convene. Team members chose to be "officers" or be the "go-to" person for decisions about components of the self-report (e.g., wording, images). This structure helped to maintain engagement as the scientists without disabilities continued to work on the self-report while awaiting additional funding. Given the relational nature of research, it is also necessary to continually evaluate the strength of team members' relationships. It can be helpful to engage in these team building practices on an ongoing basis, not only at the onset of a new collaboration. For example, when new team members join and/or long periods of time have lapsed between meetings, teams can convene for social activities.

7.4 Implications

Working to ensure people with developmental disabilities belong in science is transformative and has the potential to unearth their resiliencies and strengths, and how to leverage those for improved quality of life. Such efforts right past wrongs of abuse and exclusion, generate new knowledge poised to positively impact people with developmental disabilities, reflect disability justice, and also dramatically improve the quality of research. Research questions better reflect needed knowledge and lived realities; data collection strategies are more sensitive, accessible, and effective, thus engendering greater response rates and validity; interpretation is informed by creative implications rooted in needs, preferences, and lived experiences; and knowledge translation is more feasible and effective. Still, the positive effects of ensuring that people with developmental disabilities belong in science extends further. We found that the relationships formed between scientists with and without disabilities bear fruit that extends far beyond the research projects that bring them together. Friendships form, social capital increases, confidence and employment skills and opportunities grow, and capacity to engage in and with science expands, creating a better world for all. One example of ways that belonging to science may help individuals flourish is that an individual may start advising a research project, then serve on a grant review panel, and subsequently return to school to receive advanced scientific training (McDonald & Stack, 2016; Raymaker, 2017).

Questions for Thought and Discussion

1. Why is it important to foster the belonging of people with developmental disabilities in science?

2. What roles can researchers with disabilities assume that researchers without disabilities cannot? How do these roles benefit the research?
3. What tools and strategies can be infused in community and university settings to encourage collaborative research partnerships between those with and without disabilities?
4. What challenges are there to conducting collaborative research with researchers with disabilities?

References

Baek, K.-H., Zaslavsky, A., Lynch, R. C., Britt, C., Okada, Y., Siarey, R. J., Lensch, M. W., Park, I.-H., Yoon, S. S., Minami, T., Korenberg, J. R., Folkman, J., Daley, G. Q., Aird, W. C., Galdzicki, Z., & Ryeom, S. (2009). Down syndrome suppression of tumour growth and the role of the calcineurin inhibitor DSCR1. *Nature, 459*(7250), 1126–1130. https://doi.org/10.1038/nature08062

Bewley, C., & McCulloch, L. (2006). *Let me in-I'm a researcher: Getting involved in research.* DH Publications.

Bigby, C., Frawley, P., & Ramcharan, P. (2014). Conceptualizing inclusive research with people with intellectual disability. *Journal of Applied Research in Intellectual Disabilities, 27*(1), 3–12. https://doi.org/10.1111/jar.12083

Bottema-Beutel, K., Kapp, S. K., Lester, J. N., Sasson, N. J., & Hand, B. N. (2020). Avoiding ableist language: Suggestions for autism researchers. *Autism in Adulthood, 3*(1), 18–29. https://doi.org/10.1089/aut.2020.0014

Charlton, J. (1998). *Nothing about us without us: Disability oppression and empowerment.* University of California Press.

Clark, R. C., Nguyen, F., & Sweller, J. (2011). *Efficiency in learning: Evidence-based guidelines to manage cognitive load.* Wiley.

D'Antonio, M. (2005). *The state boys rebellion.* Simon & Schuster.

Dalton, A. J., & McVilly, K. R. (2004). Ethics guidelines for international, multicenter research involving people with intellectual disabilities. *Journal of Policy and Practice in Intellectual Disabilities, 1*(2), 57–70. https://doi.org/10.1111/j.1741-1130.2004.04010.x

Davis, L. J. (Ed.). (2013). Disability studies reader (4th ed.). Routledge.

Embregts, P., Taminiau, E., Heerkens, L., Schippers, A. P., & Van Hove, G. (2018). Collaboration in inclusive research: Competencies considered important for people with and without intellectual disabilities. *Journal of Policy and Practice in Intellectual Disabilities, 15*(3), 193–201. https://doi.org/10.1111/jppi.12248

Feldman, M. A., Bosett, J., Collet, C., & Burnham-Riosa, P. (2014). Where are persons with intellectual disabilities in medical research? A survey of published clinical trials. *Journal of Intellectual Disability Research, 58*(9), 800–809. https://doi.org/10.1111/jir.12091

Frankena, T. K., Naaldenberg, J., Cardol, M., Garcia Iriarte, E., Buchner, T., Brooker, K., Embregts, P., Joosa, E., Crowther, F., Fudge Schormans, A., Schippers, A., Walmsley, J., O'Brien, P., Linehan, C., Northway, R., van Schrojenstein Lantman-de Valk, H., & Leusink, G. (2019). A consensus statement on how to conduct inclusive health research. *Journal of Intellectual Disability Research, 63*(1), 1–11. https://doi.org/10.1111/jir.12486

Freedman, R. I. (2001). Ethical challenges in the conduct of research involving persons with mental retardation. *Mental Retardation, 39*(2), 130–141. https://doi.org/10.1352/0047-6765(2001)039<0130:ECITCO>2.0.CO;2

Garcia-Iriarte, E., Kramer, J. C., Kramer, J. M., & Hammel, J. (2009). "Who Did What?": A participatory action research project to increase group capacity for advocacy. *Journal of Applied Research in Intellectual Disabilities, 22*(1), 10–22. https://doi.org/10.1111/j.1468-3148.2008.00431.x

Garcia-Iriarte, E., O'Brien, P., McConkey, R., Wolfe, M., & O'Doherty, S. (2014). Identifying the key concerns of Irish persons with intellectual disability. *Journal of Applied Research in Intellectual Disabilities, 27*(6), 564–575. https://doi.org/10.1111/jar.12099

Habib, D. (2018). *Intelligent lives*. Like Right Now Films.

Haigh, A., Lee, D., Shaw, C., Hawthorne, M., Chamberlain, S., Newman, D. W., Clarke, Z., & Beail, N. (2013). What things make people with a learning disability happy and satisfied with their lives: An inclusive research project. *Journal of Applied Research in Intellectual Disabilities, 26*(1), 26–33. https://doi.org/10.1111/jar.12012

IACC. (2017). *2016–2017 Interagency Autism Coordinating Committee strategic plan for autism spectrum disorder*. U.S. Department of Health and Human Services Interagency Autism Coordinating Committee. https://iacc.hhs.gov/publications/strategic-plan/2017/strategic_plan_2017.pdf

Iacono, T. (2006). Ethical challenges and complexities of including people with intellectual disability as participants in research. *Journal of Intellectual & Developmental Disability, 31*(3), 173–179. https://doi.org/10.1080/13668250600876392

Inclusive Research Network. (n.d.). *How we work: The Inclusive Research Network's way of doing projects*. http://www.fedvol.ie/_fileupload/Inclusive%20Research%20Network/IRN%20How%20we%20work%20Nov2018%20final%20.pdf.

Jacobson, M. R., Azzam, T., & Baez, J. G. (2013). The nature and frequency of inclusion of people with disabilities in program evaluation. *American Journal of Evaluation, 34*(1), 23–44. https://doi.org/10.1177/1098214012461558

Jaswal, V. K., & Akhtar, N. (2018). Being vs. appearing socially uninterested: Challenging assumptions about social motivation in autism. *The Behavioral and Brain Sciences, 42*, 1–84. https://doi.org/10.1017/S0140525X18001826

Kidd, S., Davidson, L., Frederick, T., & Kral, M. J. (2018). Reflecting on participatory, action-oriented research methods in community psychology: Progress, problems, and paths forward. *American Journal of Community Psychology, 61*(1–2), 76–87. https://doi.org/10.1002/ajcp.12214

Kidney, C. A., & McDonald, K. E. (2014). A toolkit for accessible and respectful engagement in research. *Disability & Society, 29*(7), 1013–1030. https://doi.org/10.1080/09687599.2014.902357

Knox, M., Mok, M., & Parmenter, T. R. (2000). Working with the experts: Collaborative research with people with an intellectual disability. *Disability & Society, 15*(1), 49–61.

Kostanjsek, N. (2011). Use of the international classification of functioning, disability and health (ICF) as a conceptual framework and common language for disability statistics and health information systems. *BMC Public Health, 11*(S3) https://doi.org/10.1186/1471-2458-11-S4-S3

Kramer, J. M., & Schwartz, A. E. (2018). Development of the Pediatric Disability Inventory-Patient Reported Outcome (PEDI-PRO) measurement conceptual framework and item candidates. *Scandinavian Journal of Occupational Therapy, 25*(5), 335–346. https://doi.org/10.1080/11038128.2018.1502344

Kramer, J. M., Garcia-Iriarte, E., Kramer, J. C., & Hammel, J. (2011). Following through to the end: The use of inclusive strategies to analyze and interpret data in participatory action research with individuals with learning disabilities. *Journal of Applied Research in Intellectual Disabilities, 24*(3), 263–273. https://doi.org/10.1111/j.1468-3148.2010.00602.x

Kramer, J. M., Barth, Y., Curtis, K., Livingston, K., O'Neil, M., Smith, Z., Vallier, S., & Wolfe, A. (2013). Involving youth with disabilities in the development and evaluation of a new advocacy training: Project TEAM. *Disability and Rehabilitation, 35*(7), 614–622. https://doi.org/10.3109/09638288.2012.705218

Kramer, J. M., Schwartz, A. E., Watkins, D., Peace, M., Luterman, S., Barnhart, B., Bouma-Sims, J., Riley, J., Shouse, J., Maharaj, R., Rosenberg, C. R., Harvey, K., Huereña, J., Schmid, K., &

Alexander, J. S. (2019). Improving research and practice: Priorities for young adults with intellectual/developmental disabilities and mental health needs. *Journal of Mental Health Research in Intellectual Disabilities, 12*(3–4), 97–125. https://doi.org/10.1080/19315864.2019.1636910

Learning Difficulties Research Team. (2006). Let me in - I'm a researcher! Getting involved in research. The Learning Difficulties Research Team with assistance from C. Bewley and L. McCulloch: Department of Health, 116.

Lory, B. (2019). For the love of science? *Autism in Adulthood, 1*(1), 12–14. https://doi.org/10.1089/aut.2018.0005

McDonald, K. E. (2012). "We want respect": Adults with intellectual and developmental disabilities address respect in research. *American Journal on Intellectual and Developmental Disabilities, 117*(4), 263–274. https://doi.org/10.1352/1944-7558-117.4.263

McDonald, K. E., & Kidney, C. A. (2012). What is right? Ethics in intellectual disabilities research. *Journal of Policy and Practice in Intellectual Disabilities, 9*(1), 27–39. https://doi.org/10.1111/j.1741-1130.2011.00319.x

McDonald, K. E., & Raymaker, D. M. (2013). Paradigm shifts in disability and health: Toward more ethical public health research. *American Journal of Public Health, 103*(12), 2165–2173. https://doi.org/10.2105/AJPH.2013.301286

McDonald, K. E., & Stack, E. (2016). You say you want a revolution: An empirical study of community-based participatory research with people with developmental disabilities. *Disability and Health Journal, 9*(2), 201–207. https://doi.org/10.1016/j.dhjo.2015.12.006

McDonald, K. E., Kidney, C. A., & Patka, M. (2013). "You need to let your voice be heard": Research participants' views on research. *Journal of Intellectual Disability Research, 57*(3), 216–225. https://doi.org/10.1111/j.1365-2788.2011.01527.x

McDonald, K. E., Conroy, N., Olick, R., Kim, C., LaBraico, E., Prother, E., & The Project ETHICS Expert Panel. (2016a). Is safety in the eye of the beholder? Safeguards in research with adults with intellectual disability. *Journal of Empirical Research in Human Research Ethics, 11*, 424–438. https://doi.org/10.1177/1556264616651182

McDonald, K. E., Conroy, N., Olick, R. S., & Project ETHICS Expert Panel. (2016b). Is it worth it? Benefits in research with adults with intellectual disability. *Intellectual and Developmental Disabilities, 54*, 440–453. https://doi.org/10.1352/1934-9556-54.6.440

McDonald, K. E., Fialka-Feldman, M., Barkoff, A., & Burgdorf, M. (2020). Legal, ethical, and social issues affecting the lives of people with intellectual and developmental disabilities. In A. L. M. Glidden, L. L. McIntyre, & M. J. Tasse (Eds.), *American Psychological Association handbook on intellectual and developmental disabilities*. American Psychological Association.

Milner, P., & Frawley, P. (2018). From 'on' to 'with' to 'by:' People with a learning disability creating a space for the third wave of inclusive research. *Qualitative Research, 19*(4), 382–398. https://doi.org/10.1177/1468794118781385

Morgan, M. F., Moni, K. B., & Cuskelly, M. (2015). The development of research skills in young adults with intellectual disability in participatory research. *International Journal of Disability, Development, and Education, 62*(4), 438–457. https://doi.org/10.1080/1034912X.2015.1028905

National Commission for the Protection of Human Subjects of Biomedical and Behavioral Research. (1979). *Belmont report: Ethical principles and guidelines for the protection of human subjects of research*. U.S. Department of Health and Human Services. https://www.hhs.gov/ohrp/regulations-and-policy/belmont-report/read-the-belmont-report/index.html

National Institutes of Health. (2009). *Research involving individuals with questionable capacity to consent: Points to consider*. http://grants.nih.gov/grants/policy/questionablecapacity.htm.

Nelson, L. L. (this volume). Using the Universal Design for Learning framework to understand the power of belonging. In J. L. Jones & K. L. Gallus (Vol. Eds.), *Belonging and resilience in individuals with intellectual and developmental disabilities – Community and family engagement*. Springer.

Neudel, E. (2011). *Lives worth living*. Storyline Motion Pictures & Independent Television Service.

Nicolaidis, C. (2012). What can physicians learn from the neurodiversity movement? *The Virtual Mentor: VM, 14*(6), 503–510. https://doi.org/10.1001/virtualmentor.2012.14.6.oped1-1206

Nicolaidis, C., Raymaker, D., McDonald, K., Dern, S., Ashkenazy, E., Boisclair, C., Robertson, S., & Baggs, A. (2011). Collaboration strategies in nontraditional community-based participatory research partnerships: Lessons from an academic–community partnership with autistic self-advocates. *Progress in Community Health Partnerships, 5*(2), 143–150. https://doi.org/10.1353/cpr.2011.0022

Nicolaidis, C., Raymaker, D., Katz, M., Oschwald, M., Goe, R., Leotti, S., Grantham, L., Plourde, E., Salomon, J., Hughes, R. B., & Partnering with People with Disabilities to Address Violence Consortium. (2015). Community-based participatory research to adapt health measures for use by people with developmental disabilities. *Progress in Community Health Partnerships: Research, Education, and Action, 9*(2), 157–170. https://doi.org/10.1353/cpr.2015.0037

Nicolaidis, C., Raymaker, D., Kapp, S. K., Baggs, A., Ashkenazy, E., McDonald, K., Weiner, M., Maslak, J., Hunter, M., & Joyce, A. (2019). The AASPIRE practice-based guidelines for the inclusion of autistic adults in research as co-researchers and study participants. *Autism: The International Journal of Research and Practice, 23*(8), 2007–2019. https://doi.org/10.1177/1362361319830523

Nicolaidis, C., Raymaker, D., McDonald, K., Lund, E., Leotti, S., Knapp, M., Katz, M., Beers, L., Kripke, C., Maslak, J., Hunter, M., & Zhen, K. (2020). Creating accessible survey instruments for use with autistic adults and people with intellectual disability: Lessons learned and recommendations. *Autism in Adulthood, 2*(1), 61–76. https://doi.org/10.1089/aut.2019.0074

Nind, M., & Vinha, H. (2012). Doing research inclusively: Bridges to multiple possibilities in inclusive research. *British Journal of Learning Disabilities, 42*(2), 102–109. https://doi.org/10.1111/bld.12013

Northway, R. (2014). To include or not to include? That is the ethical question. *Journal of Intellectual Disabilities, 18*(3), 209–210. https://doi.org/10.1177/1744629514543863

Northway, R., Hurley, K., O'Connor, C., Thomas, H., Howarth, J., Langley, E., & Bale, S. (2014). Deciding what to research: An overview of a participatory workshop. *British Journal of Learning Disabilities, 42*(4), 323–327. https://doi.org/10.1111/bld.12080

O'Brien, P., McConkey, R., & García-Iriarte, E. (2014). Co-researching with people who have intellectual disabilities: Insights from a national survey. *Journal of Applied Research in Intellectual Disabilities, 27*(1), 65–75. https://doi.org/10.1111/jar.12074

Office of Autism Research Coordination, National Institute of Mental Health, Autistica, Canadian Institutes of, Health Research, & Macquarie University. (2019). *2016 International autism spectrum disorder research portfolio analysis report*. U.S. Department of Health and Human Services Interagency Autism Coordinating Committee. https://iacc.hhs.gov/publications/international-portfolio-analysis/2016

Oliver, M. (1990). *The politics of disablement: A sociological approach*. St. Martin's Press.

Raymaker, D. M. (2017). Reflections of a community-based participatory researcher from the intersection of disability advocacy, engineering, and the academy. *Action Research, 15*(3), 258–275. https://doi.org/10.1177/1476750316636669

Salmon, N., Barry, A., & Hutchins, E. (2018). Inclusive research: An Irish perspective. *British Journal of Learning Disabilities, 46*(4), 268–277. https://doi.org/10.1111/bld.12247

Schwartz, A. E., & Durkin, B. (2020). "Team is everything": Reflections on trust, logistics, and methodological choices in collaborative interviewing. *British Journal of Learning Disabilities*. https://doi.org/10.1111/bld.12305

Schwartz, A. E., Kramer, J. M., Cohn, E. S., & McDonald, K. E. (2020a). "That felt like real engagement": Fostering and maintaining inclusive research collaborations with individuals with intellectual disability. *Qualitative Health Research, 30*(2), 236–249. https://doi.org/10.1177/1049732319869620

Schwartz, A. E., Kramer, J. M., & PEDI-PRO Youth Team. (2020b). Inclusive approaches to developing content valid patient-reported outcome measure response scales for youth with intellectual/developmental disabilities. *British Journal of Learning Disabilities*. https://doi.org/10.1111/bld.12346

Schwartz, A. E., Young Adult Mental Health/Peer Mentoring Research, Kramer, J. M., Rogers, E. S., McDonald, K. E., & Cohn, E. S. (2020c). Stakeholder-driven approach to developing a peer-mentoring intervention for young adults with intellectual/developmental disabilities and co-occurring mental health conditions. *Journal of Applied Research in Intellectual Disabilities, 33*(5), 992–1004. https://doi.org/10.1111/jar.12721

Seekins, T., & White, G. W. (2012). Participatory action research designs in applied disability and rehabilitation science: Protecting against threats to social validity. *Archives of Physical Medicine and Rehabilitation, 94*(1), S20–S29. https://doi.org/10.1016/j.apmr.2012.07.033

Spong, C. Y., & Bianchi, D. W. (2018). Improving public health requires inclusion of underrepresented populations in research. *JAMA, 319*(4), 337–338. https://doi.org/10.1001/jama.2017.19138

Stack, E., & McDonald, K. E. (2014). Nothing about us without us: Does action research in developmental disabilities research measure up? *Journal of Policy and Practice in Intellectual Disabilities, 11*(2), 83–91. https://doi.org/10.1111/jppi.12074

Stack, E., & McDonald, K. E. (2018). We are "both in charge, the academics and self-advocates": Empowerment in community-based participatory research. *Journal of Policy and Practice in Intellectual Disabilities, 15*(1), 80–89. https://doi.org/10.1111/jppi.12236

Straus, S. E., Tetroe, J., & Graham, I. (2009). Defining knowledge translation. *CMAJ: Canadian Medical Association Journal, 181*(3–4), 165–168. https://doi.org/10.1503/cmaj.081229

Strnadová, I., & Walmsley, J. (2018). Peer-reviewed articles on inclusive research: Do co-researchers with intellectual disabilities have a voice? *Journal of Applied Research in Intellectual Disabilities, 31*(1), 132–141. https://doi.org/10.1111/jar.12378

Strnadova, I., Walmsley, J., Johnson, K., & Cumming, T. M. (2016). Diverse faces of inclusive research: Reflecting on three research studies. *Scandinavian Journal of Disability Research, 18*(1), 52–64. https://doi.org/10.1080/15017419.2014.964766

Walmsley, J. (2004). Inclusive learning disability research: The (nondisabled) researcher's role. *British Journal of Learning Disabilities, 32*, 65–71. https://doi.org/10.1111/j.1468-3156.2004.00281.x

Walmsley, J., Strnadova, I., & Johnson, K. (2018). The added value of inclusive research. *Journal of Applied Research in Intellectual Disabilities, 31*(5), 751–759. https://doi.org/10.1111/jar.12431

Zarb, G. (1992). On the road to Damascus: First steps towards changing the relations of disability research production. *Disability, Handicap, & Society, 7*(2), 125–138. https://doi.org/10.1080/02674649266780161

Chapter 8
Belonging and Inclusion: Supporting Individuals and Families Throughout the Future Planning Process

Lynne T. Tomasa and Heather J. Williamson

Future planning is the process where an individual with intellectual and developmental disabilities (IDD), their family, and network of support begin to create a plan that guides every aspect of their daily life. It includes difficult conversations about the transition of caregiving roles, residential or living arrangements, finances, decision-making supports, social engagement, relationships, and necessary supports. Future planning minimizes confusion and increases the likelihood that individuals with IDD can continue to achieve their personal goals when their primary supports, or social environments change.

The chapter highlights the societal and support needs that an aging America must address to ensure that individuals can continue to actively participate in decision-making and families can plan for their futures. Additional topics related to future planning are presented as we move toward understanding the lives of four families working on their future plans. Carter's (2016) model of belonging is used to show how individuals with IDD and families can engage each other during the planning process and how belonging enhances resilience within families and communities.

L. T. Tomasa (✉)
Sonoran Center for Excellence in Disabilities, Department of Family and Community Medicine, University of Arizona, Tucson, AZ, USA
e-mail: ltomasa@arizona.edu

H. J. Williamson
Center for Health Equity Research, Department of Occupational Therapy, Northern Arizona University, Flagstaff, AZ, USA

J. L. Jones, K. L. Gallus (eds.), *Belonging and Resilience in Individuals with Developmental Disabilities*, Emerging Issues in Family and Individual Resilience, https://doi.org/10.1007/978-3-030-81277-5_8

8.1 The Socio-ecological Framework as a Way to Understand Future Planning

The socio-ecological framework is a useful lens to understand the complexity of the future planning process. Bronfenbrenner (1977) brought attention to how individuals develop through the lifespan and interact within and between different ecological systems that include their families, communities, and the broader society in which they reside. The ecological framework has been applied broadly in the disability field, including to examine quality of life and planning for older adults with autism (Edelson et al., 2021). During the future planning process, the socio-ecological approach can explain how the interrelationships among individual characteristics and experiences, relationships, settings, communities, and societal factors can influence conversations, decision-making, and outcomes for individuals with IDD and their families.

8.1.1 Demographics of an Aging Society

There is a demographic shift occurring in the United States. Future projections anticipate that persons over 65 will go from 49 million in 2016 to 95 million in 2060 and the number of people 85 and older will nearly triple by 2060 (Vespa et al., 2020). Unlike caring for older parents, aging family caregivers often provide support and day-to-day care for a family member with IDD over the course of their lives. These families are challenged to balance caregiving and their own personal needs. In addition to an aging society, individuals with IDD are living longer lives requiring longer duration of support from family caregivers. In developed countries, individuals with IDD are living into their 60s, as compared to 30–35 years in the 1970–1980s (Dolan et al., 2019). By 2030, it has been projected that there will be 1.4 million people with IDD over the age of 60 in the United States (Factor et al., 2012). Factors contributing to longer life expectancies of people with IDD include advances in health care, changes in the mechanism by which services and supports are provided (including moving from institutional-based services to home and community-based services), and providing more individualized supports (Haley & Perkins, 2004; Ervin et al., 2014).

8.1.2 Existing Disparities Among Individuals with Intellectual and Developmental Disabilities

Although there is a notable extension in the longevity of life among adults with IDD, significant disparities exist compared to their peers without disabilities including higher rates of chronic disease (National Academies of Science, Engineering, and Medicine, 2018). The lack of inclusion in health promotion programs and lack of access to care contribute to the health disparities experienced by adults with IDD (U. S. Department of Health and Human Services, 2005). Latino and Black adults with IDD have worse health outcomes (Magaña, et al., 2016). Those who identify as non-White have more unmet service needs, are less likely to see a general practitioner, and are less likely to receive dental care (Scott & Havercamp, 2014; Burke & Heller, 2017). Aging adults with IDD have fewer financial resources, less access to health care, and more limited social supports outside of their family unit as compared to their younger counterparts (Heller et al., 2010).

8.1.3 Family Caregivers

Currently, there are more than one in five Americans or approximately 21% who are providing care to a loved one with a disability and among them, 16.8% of caregivers are 50 years and older (AARP & National Alliance for Caregiving, 2020). For persons with IDD, approximately 70% of individuals are living with a family caregiver, and among these caregivers 24% are age 60 years or older (Tanis et al., 2020). Family caregivers provide both instrumental (i.e., activities of daily living, instrumental activities of daily living) and emotional supports for their loved one, yet their needs are not systematically addressed in existing service systems (Williamson & Perkins, 2014). Aging family caregivers of adults with IDD report reduced well-being and more declines in health compared to parents of adults without disabilities (Namkung et al., 2018). Compared to the general population, aging family caregivers of individuals with IDD who share the same home had higher prevalence of high blood pressure, arthritis, obesity, and activities of daily living limitations (Yamaki et al., 2009). If family caregivers feel that they are giving more support than they are receiving from their loved one with IDD (disadvantage of reciprocity), then they report poor mental health (Perkins & Haley, 2013).

There are also beneficial experiences related to being a family caregiver of an individual with IDD. The caregiving role for parents is considered a normative role, in that it is a normal role expectation to care for a child as opposed to caring for a spouse or a parent (Haley & Perkins, 2004). Additionally, family caregivers of individuals with IDD are often providing care over the life course which can allow them to develop expertise and feelings of mastery in their caregiving role (Haley & Perkins, 2004). When aging family caregivers of adults with IDD engage in problem-solving and finding solutions, they demonstrate improved resiliency and reduced caregiver burden (Piazza et al., 2014).

8.1.4 Context of Aging in Future Planning

The longevity of the older population including adults with IDD places increasing demands on families and service systems. Alongside these demands is the need to plan for the futures of caregivers, care recipients, and family units. Lakin and Burke (2019) present six issues that are important to address for aging persons with severe disabilities and persons who develop severe disabilities as they age: (a) transitioning to retirement, (b) finding and securing appropriate services and supports, (c) ensuring continued support from family and friends, (d) sustaining a healthy lifestyle in order to have optimal health, (e) addressing grief and end-of-life issues, and (f) recognizing the importance of friendships as it relates to loneliness and isolation. These issues impact the quality of life for individuals with IDD, particularly as they age alongside family members and peers. For families who are looking toward the future, addressing these issues can be an overwhelming challenge as parents plan for themselves as well as for their child with a disability.

8.2 Future Planning: Research

8.2.1 Multidimensional Aspects of Future Planning

The research on future planning spans more than 30 years and continues to be an important topic for individuals with IDD, family members, service providers, policy makers, and researchers. Future planning consists of complex and often emotional decisions that present over time or at different transition points for families. Decisions focus on ensuring and protecting the quality of life for individuals with IDD. The following literature provides an overview of key aspects of the future planning process.

Aging family caregivers worry that their family member with IDD may outlive them and must determine options for alternatives to long-term care for their loved one. One important consideration is the current and future living arrangements for individuals with IDD. In the United States in 2017, an estimated 72% of 7,416,011 persons with IDD lived with a family caregiver with the remainder living alone with a roommate (18%) or in a supervised residential setting (10%). Of those living with family caregivers, 41% of the caregivers were younger than 41 years of age, 35% were age 41 to 59, and 24% were 60 and older (Tanis et al., 2020).

The focus of future planning is on creating a plan that represents the wishes and goals of the person with IDD and engages them as much as possible during the planning process. Future planning is a process by which individuals with IDD and relevant family members discuss and make decisions about where to live, getting a job, managing finances, making decisions, having relationships, and engaging with their community (The Arc Center for Future Planning, n.d.). The emphasis is on building a support network so a person can be as independent as possible. End of life planning is not typically listed as a formal part of a plan but can be integrated in health care and legal planning documents such as advance directives and special needs trusts. Future planning can be a helpful process for identifying what types of supports will be necessary when the long-term caregiver (i.e., parent or sibling) is not available or able to provide support. A lack of thoughtful planning can have negative consequences if sudden and undesirable transitions occur. For example, without timely planning, adults with IDD may be transferred to an inappropriate institutional setting and new care providers will be unaware of the person's unique needs, abilities, and preferences (Hewitt et al., 2010).

Lindahl et al. (2019) interviewed parents and siblings of adults with IDD and identified the following planning domains: housing and living arrangements, legal planning, identification of a primary caregiver, financial planning, daily care, management of medical issues, and transportation coordination. Brief descriptions of the domains are presented next. Housing and living arrangements were seen as one of the most important domains and included the option of living in a group home, with relatives, or independent living. Legal planning involved transferring legal power of attorney, sharing co-guardianship, and designating someone if a guardian was necessary in the future. Families also identified one or more future primary caregivers that would share responsibilities and serve as a network of support. The financial domain overlapped with the legal domain when it involved a special needs trust, life insurance, will, or Medicaid funding. Managing financial costs were viewed as a barrier to planning. Day-to-day care and activities included finding and managing care providers, planning for chores and maintenance, and finding day programs or employment opportunities. Medical management can be a complicated area as medical care and needs increase. Planning for transportation involved having an accessible vehicle and having someone to drive to and from medical appointments, jobs, and activities. The identification of a primary caregiver, who may also be the designated guardian, was often a first step in facilitating planning (Lindahl et al., 2019).

Anderson et al. (2018) found that over 50% of caregivers of individuals with IDD did not have a plan for the future and caregivers from lower socioeconomic backgrounds were less likely to report a future plan than those from higher socioeconomic backgrounds. Family caregivers expressed concerns about planning for the future but often lacked the necessary services and supports to help navigate the future planning process (Dillenburger & McKerr, 2011; Ryan et al., 2014). Parental caregivers know that future planning is necessary but often cannot anticipate when to start the process (Tomasa & Shirai, 2008). Caregivers reported the following experiences that served as facilitators or barriers to planning: (a) person with IDD's desire for increased independence; (b) caregiver exhaustion, inability to continue, or death; (c) family and friends encouraging a change as beneficial to both the parent and child; (d) negative experiences with institutions; (e) growing dependence between caregiver and care recipient; (f) and concern about the safety and well-being of their family member while in the care of others (Tomasa & Shirai, 2008).

The quality of life of aging individuals with IDD is likely to improve if they engage in future planning efforts (Schepens et al., 2019). Individuals with IDD may be involved with decision-making in various ways. For example, those involved in the planning process were more likely to make decisions about leisure activities rather than formal decisions regarding daily supports (Burke et al., 2019). The planning process involves supporting the individual to self-determine their future wishes, while also balancing the perspectives of family members (Hewitt et al., 2013). In examining the planning process, it is important to understand the potential barriers to planning.

8.2.2 Barriers to Future Planning

There are various factors that may hinder the planning process. Walker and Hutchinson (2018) reported that among older parents, a combination of internal and external barriers influenced the completion of a plan. For example, there were family dynamics or events that prompted the making of plans and families varied regarding their readiness to plan. The findings suggest that parents need support in the planning process and a "one size approach" does not work (Walker & Hutchinson, 2018).

A review by Bibby (2013) identified ten factors that serve as barriers to future planning. The barriers were identified as: (a) lack of confidence in present and future provision, (b) difficult relationship with professionals, (c) mutual care and interdependency, (d) lack of information, (e) painful/difficult subject, (f) carer purpose and identity, (g) carer sense of duty, (h) fear of the unknown, (i) carer concern regarding loss of control, and (j) service-user unwilling to leave home. In a 2015 web-based survey, the barriers identified by parents included the lack of appropriate services (residential, employment, and recreational support), financial concerns, lack of information, reluctance or refusal of family members to participate in planning, time, difficult emotions, lack of motivation, and no family member to succeed as caregiver. The most prevalent barrier was the lack of available services and its fragmented service system (Burke et al., 2018). Owen et al. (2020) asked professionals to identify the barriers they felt families experienced and the barriers they experienced as professionals working with individuals and families. Professionals identified family barriers in order of frequency as the (a) lack of information, (b) lack of financial resources, (c) lack of options in the community, (d) familial fears about end-of-life issues, and (e) family conflict. As a professional, they identified the top two most frequent barriers as lack of knowledge about the same issues as families and lack of community options. This was followed by family conflict, lack of time to spend with each family, difficulty in assessing the choices and desires of the person with IDD, confusion about the meaning of person-centered planning, unsupportive organizational policies and practices, and inadequate organizational commitment (Owen et al., 2020).

8.2.3 *Interpersonal Relationships: The Role of Siblings in Future Planning*

The role of siblings as caregivers is an emerging area of research. Siblings often anticipate and assume more significant roles in the future. They serve as advocates in a formal or legal capacity, mediator with systems of care, supervisor of daily living activities, and provider of direct care. They are also likely to oversee the well-being of their sibling with IDD in the future. Siblings may be involved in future planning alongside their sibling with IDD but may experience challenges if they have conflicting views from their parents (Lee et al., 2019a). Coyle et al. (2014) explored the perspectives of 16 siblings over the age of 60 as they became the primary caregiver for an adult with IDD. Balancing their sibling's needs with their family needs was a challenge, and it was less stressful if parents made plans and communicated expectations before the actual transition occurred. Lee et al. (2019b) conducted interviews with ten parent-sibling dyads and identified future planning barriers that were family related, systemic, and related to the person with IDD. Family communication was often superficial and planning activities lacked specificity. Parents and siblings reported financial concerns and the lack of systemic supports. Parents reported the vulnerability of people with IDD as a barrier while siblings reported balancing their own lives as a barrier (Lee et al., 2019b).

It is easy to view planning as a set of steps, tasks, or responsibilities instead of focusing on the sibling relationship. Parents and siblings can find it difficult to approach the topic of future planning with each other and may have conflicting ideas about what is best for the individual with IDD. The individual may also have their own ideas that don't align with their parents or siblings (Rossetti et al., 2020). For example, parents may focus on keeping the individual safe and having consistent supports while siblings may be more comfortable taking risks and focusing on quality of life (Rossetti et al., 2020).

8.2.4 *Person-Centered Planning and Supported Decision-Making in Future Planning*

To the best of their ability, individuals with IDD can and should be encouraged to actively engage in the planning of their futures. They can do this by having a central role in creating a team or network of individuals that support their desire to engage in the community and live as independently as possible. Person-centered planning (PCP) practices have been used and advocated for with adults with IDD as an approach to identify individual strengths, create a vision for the future, and encourage choice in supports, services, and daily life activities (The Arc, 2018). In an effort to address long-term services and supports, the National Quality Forum (2020) brought together stakeholders and published an updated definition of

PCP. The definition is written in plain language and directed toward the person. The person-first definition states,

> Person-centered planning is an approach to support you in living the kind of life you want for yourself. The plan includes organizing your supports and services. You are able to explore all areas of life that are important to you. You can choose to make a plan with the support of people you are close to. You decide the kinds of supports and services you need. You also decide how to organize them in a way that works for you. You are in charge of the meetings. You decide who comes to the meetings. You decide where and when they happen. This type of planning goes on for the entire time you use support. You can change any part of the plan you want at any time. It is not done just during a planning meeting. Decisions are usually made in a meeting or a series of meetings. (p. 8)

The person-centered planning process can be influenced by external factors including the capacity of the care recipient, family, and support services (McCausland et al., 2019).

Supported decision-making (SDM) builds on the person-centered planning process, focuses on identifying supports needed for decision-making, and enhances self-determination (Shogren et al., 2017). It is the understanding that everyone has the right to make choices and each person may need different types of support in making decisions (National Resource Center for Supported Decision-Making, n.d.). Supported decision-making involves creating a network that includes people they trust who can help understand potential issues, situations, and choices by using language that is understood by the individual with IDD (Whitlatch & Ullman, 2020). It is the least restrictive alternative to guardianship. It does not require a legal petition, is a fluid process, and does not impose potential long-term limitations on an individual's rights, personal liberties, and choices.

Campanella (2015) identifies key concepts critical to the understanding of SDM. They include: (a) life experiences allow individuals to develop the capacity for decision-making; (b) support teams need to learn about each person's unique abilities and desires; (c) the process is not always easy or risk free; (d) the role of support is to stay focused on what the person wants; (e) the capacity for decision-making is not static and can change over time due to skill building and accumulated experiences; and (f) the role of direct support professionals and service organizations can shift to being a coach that allows the person with IDD to lead.

Shogren and Wehmeyer (2015) use the socio-ecological model of disability as a framework for understanding SDM as a personalized process that changes over the life course. The framework consisted of three domains: contextual factors, environmental demands, and supports needed. At the individual level, supporting decision-making requires understanding personal characteristics, skills, and knowledge. Environmental demands include the decisions needed to address health and medical issues. The identification of needed supports requires understanding a person's abilities. In a synthesis of the literature, Shogren et al. (2017) identified categories of contextual (personal) and environmental factors and demands that influence decision-making. Contextual categories included sociodemographic characteristics, decision-making experience, co-occurring conditions, and emotional factors.

Environmental demands included accessibility of information, complexity of decision, relationships with providers, living arrangement, opportunities for decision-making, and family attitudes about decision-making.

8.2.5 Interventions and Models to Support Future Planning

Various strategies and models to support individuals with IDD and families with future planning activities have been identified. Group interventions have been shown to be successful in providing information and support to families. Six-week group psychoeducational interventions provided parents with information and resources about planning and opportunities to interact with other parents ultimately leading to increased confidence and competence to plan (Smith et al., 1996; Botsford & Rule, 2004). The *Future is Now* curriculum is based on a model of peer support for individuals with IDD and their adult relatives who want to learn about and participate in future planning activities. Individuals with IDD and family members meet together and then break out into separate peer groups to address future dreams, support networks, living arrangements, work, education, retirement, and strategies to assure that their future plan will be implemented. Families are provided training on legal and financial aspects of planning (Heller & Caldwell, 2006). Planning activities can also occur in community settings with service providers. For example, a brief transition-of-care form served as an introduction to future planning at an adult habilitation agency (Tencza & Forsythe, 2019). The form was a useful way to share information about the direction individuals with IDD wanted their life to go if their current situation changed. In a multistate intervention, professionals attended a one-day educational and skill-building training where participants reported feeling more confident about their knowledge and ability to support families and individuals with IDD through the future planning process (Owen et al., 2020). The Arc Center for Future Planning also has an online tool that is designed for individuals with IDD, family, friends, and professional staff to participate in building a plan by creating an account within the Center. The online tool provides information on the following areas: expressing wishes for the future, deciding where to live, financing the future, employment and daily activities, supporting daily and major life decisions, and making social connections.

The research on future planning identified the multidimensional influences on future planning for adults with IDD and their families. Considering the importance of completing future plans, more research is needed on interventions to support siblings and how individuals with IDD participate and contribute to the planning process (Lee & Burke, 2020). In the next section, reflections on future planning will be shared through the experiences of families who actively engaged in the process.

8.3 Future Planning: Worksheets and Case Examples

The *Future Planning: A Roadmap of Our Futures Our Wishes* (Tomasa, 2018) is a workbook that was developed to facilitate communication and planning. It is based on actual experiences from interviews with individuals with IDD and their families. It recognizes that risks, choices, and emotions are an important part of the discussions. Future planning is a process that involves getting to know the individual, involving them in all aspects of planning, maintaining and building new relationships, clarifying expectations and roles, and adjusting plans as different life events occur. By having open and honest conversations, professionals can create a sense of belonging and support individual and family resilience.

The *Future Planning: A Roadmap of Our Futures Our Wishes* (Tomasa, 2018) consists of four chapters. Chapter one talks about planning as a journey; chapter two consists of worksheets that introduce important conversations; chapter three consists of additional topics to explore; and chapter four shares personal stories. The emphasis here is on chapter two which consists of 14 worksheets, each with a different focus and purpose. The worksheets are designed to facilitate conversations that may be difficult and provides a space to share ideas or a checklist of items to discuss. Individuals with IDD, family members, or people who provide support can choose worksheets that apply to their personal situation. It is not necessary to complete all of them, and worksheets do not have to be completed in a particular order. The worksheets can be done separately by each individual and then shared with each other or worked on together.

Two of the 14 worksheets are presented in Table 8.1. The roadmap can be downloaded, and permission is granted to reprint all or parts of the workbook to be used for the purpose of future planning.

The following narratives provide insight from four families regarding their experiences with future planning. It is important to recognize that planning is fluid and decisions can change based on individual, family, and environmental contexts. Plans should be revisited and updated regularly.

8.3.1 Jim and Ann (Mother)

Jim is a 42-year-old gentleman with IDD who loves to watch YouTube videos and the weather channel. His older brother Lyle lives in another state with his wife. Jim's mother Ann is his guardian, and they talk openly about their futures. Jim was living with his father until his death, moved to a townhouse next to his mother, and now lives with his mother who is 67 years old. He was active with Special Olympics until he had an injury. Jim has been employed at the same place for the last 15 years. He participates in a day program and attends weekly church services. He is a very social person and has many friends. Jim and his mother have always talked openly about their futures and together they discuss the pros and cons of their decisions. At

Table 8.1 Example worksheets for future planning

Worksheet	Purpose and use
This is Me and My Life (page 23) 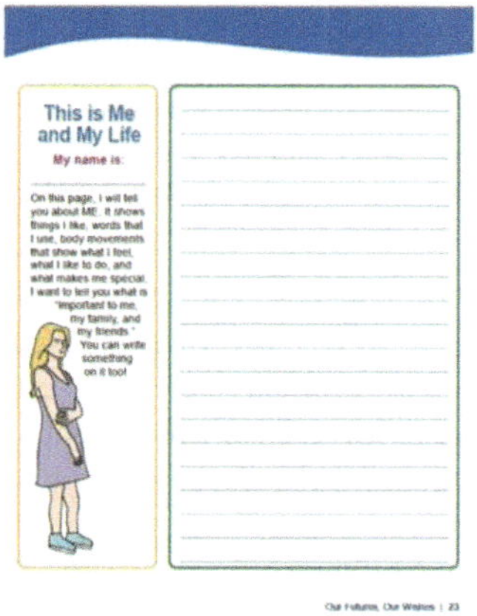 This is Me and My Life My name is: On this page, I will tell you about ME. It shows things I like, words that I use, body movements that show what I feel, what I like to do, and what makes me special. I want to tell you what is "important to me, my family, and my friends." You can write something on it too! Our Futures, Our Wishes | 23	*This is Me and My Life* is a one-page worksheet that takes a person-centered approach by providing individuals with IDD an opportunity to talk about themselves and their life. The focus is on what is important to them. This worksheet can be used to facilitate getting to know the individual and invite others to participate in the conversation. It is helpful when introducing new support providers, updating family, or when joining a new social situation. It encourages a sense of belonging.
Circle of Support: Self-Assessment Checklist 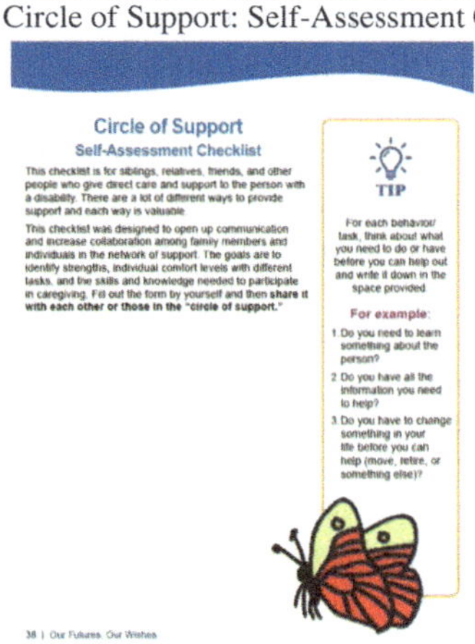 Circle of Support Self-Assessment Checklist This checklist is for siblings, relatives, friends, and other people who give direct care and support to the person with a disability. There are a lot of different ways to provide support and each way is valuable. This checklist was designed to open up communication and increase collaboration among family members and individuals in the network of support. The goals are to identify strengths, individual comfort levels with different tasks, and the skills and knowledge needed to participate in caregiving. Fill out the form by yourself and then **share it with each other or those in the "circle of support."** TIP For each behavior/task, think about what you need to do or have before you can help out and write it down in the space provided. For example: 1. Do you need to learn something about the person? 2. Do you have all the information you need to help? 3. Do you have to change something in your life before you can help (move, retire, or something else)? 38 | Our Futures, Our Wishes	*Circle of Support: Self-Assessment Checklist* is a five-page worksheet designed to assess and build a person's network of support. The focus is on minimizing conflict and confusion among individuals who provide support by clarifying roles and expectations. The worksheet can be used to form collaborations and to identify the type and degree of support someone can provide. There are four pages of behaviors and tasks that address relationships, activities of daily living, employment, health, finances, and legal and supportive decision-making.

Note. Adapted and printed with permission from Tomasa, L. (2018). *Future planning: A Roadmap of Our Futures Our Wishes*. Sonoran Center for Excellence in Disabilities. https://sonoranucedd.fcm.arizona.edu/publications/OurFuturesOurWishes

one point, Jim's plan was to move to Texas to live with his brother and his wife who is a special education teacher. This seemed like an ideal plan until Jim saw a tornado on the news where his brother lives. Jim no longer wanted to move there after seeing the devastation it caused.

Jim experienced several changes to his usual routine. Due to the increase in the minimum wage, Jim had to reduce his employment to one day a week in order to continue to qualify for his government benefits. The coronavirus (COVID-19) pandemic forced Jim and his mother to look for different ways to stay connected since they were isolated in their home. During this period of social isolation, he decided to retire from his long-time job (15 years) and participate only in his day program when it reopened. This made Jim and his mother reflect on what life would be like if he remained alone in Tucson or moved to Dallas to be close to his brother.

> I (mother) have been trying to decide myself just how important "belonging" is to quality of life. If Jim were here in Tucson without family, I think it is possible that the lack of a safety net in the form of family might negate the value of "belonging" somewhat. Old friends are wonderful, but they too get sick and might be unable to be much support. He would be vulnerable here in Tucson alone. Moving to Dallas would be difficult, but he could make new friends through a new church and Special Olympics.

Jim once had a 10-day visit with his brother and sister-in-law. The time together allowed everyone to experience what it might look like to live together. It became clear that each person had established their own lives and routines in different cities and that they will need to get reacquainted on a personal level. Lyle needs to understand how Jim spends his time, what his interests and strengths are, and what type of supports he needs. Jim and Lyle will need to create new networks of supports for each of them. Ann told her son and daughter-in-law during their visit to see Jim that an ideal arrangement would include, "An apartment, if you can give him a lot of independence, I think his quality of life will be better rather than trying to have everything totally sheltered…. See what he can do, let him have as much as he can safely have."

Ann believes that Jim is fairly resilient and "if someone is truly happy and stable, that makes them more resilient in the long run." Plans will likely change, but at the core of planning is an understanding of who the person is. Worksheets within the *Future Planning: A Roadmap of Our Future Our Wishes* that could assist Jim during this time include (1) This is Me and My Life, (2) This is Me and Our Lives, and (3) Things or Activities That Bring Me Joy and Make Me Feel Good. Transitions to a new community or residential living arrangement can be difficult if assumptions are made by family members. Transitions can be better facilitated by an understanding that each person had their own routines, likes, and friendships that define what makes a good and meaningful life. *Future Planning* worksheets can help to open up that conversation. While the plan is for Lyle to become Jim's guardian, guardianship does not negate an exploration or the importance of supported decision-making.

8.3.2 Rebecca the "Dancing Queen" and Mary (Mother)

Rebecca is a 37-year-old woman who lives with her parents Mary and Joe, both in their 70s. She has a rare genetic disorder and an intellectual disability. Rebecca is fondly known as "Dancing Queen" by her friends because she loves music and dancing. Her three older siblings moved away for college and work. Sister Suzi recently returned to town and lives nearby. Dancing Queen communicates using short phrases on her augmentative communication device (AAC) which required extensive paperwork to get approval and coverage by her health insurance. She participates in activities through The Arc, Special Olympics, church, and AAC group. According to Mary, "Our pastor measures how well the parish is doing on how well they treat Rebecca." In 2007, Mary had a conversation with her children about how they were going to be involved in Rebecca's life in the future. Ten years later, she realized that "we're going to have to keep talking to the other kids as their life changes to make sure that what we thought and what they said they were going to do is actually going to happen." Mary also realized that their roles as caregivers are changing.

> There is more to being a caregiver. One has to come up with goals and objectives, do the annuals, do the meetings, go to doctor appointments, complete paperwork, ... I realized that as we're getting older, we have to take a more active role of getting them (siblings) trained to understand how to work with Rebecca.

Each of the siblings will have a specific role based on their knowledge and comfort with certain tasks or responsibilities. For example, Lily will be in charge of the trust and Suzi will be the payee and day-to-day caregiver. John has his own family, so his role will be to provide respite for Suzi and to stay socially connected as much as he can. During this transition of roles, Mary reflected that, "it is difficult for Suzi to understand that she is not just her sister, but she is somebody that has to allow Rebecca to have her independence." Mary and Joe have made financial and legal plans that will allow the siblings to take trips together. One suggestion Mary has for others is to have a person-centered plan.

> It (person-centered plan) has really forced us to carry out what Rebecca wants to do. The plan is reviewed regularly several times a year.... It takes a lot of time and thought to put together a good plan because you really have to listen and do what is important to the individual.

Mary also has a suggestion for working with systems. She wants individuals who are at a planning meeting to ask the right questions.

> Instead of asking, how are your services? What are her health care needs? Have the medicines changed? This does not capture who they were in the 90 days since the team last reviewed Dancing Queen's person-centered plan. One should ask, Who did she see? Where did she go? What did she like? What were some of her health care needs?

As a family, Mary believes that parents must have high expectations and "remove the barriers." For example, Rebecca enjoys golfing with her parents. Her father called the city officials who later changed their policy to allow people with IDD to ride in the cart with another person. *Future Planning* worksheets recommended for Rebecca and her family include (1) Pieces of Our Plan and (2) Circle of Support. The Pieces of Our Plan worksheet identifies the domains or general areas in a person's plan. Not all areas need to be addressed at the same time. It serves as a starting point for conversations about future planning. The Circle of Support worksheet is a self-assessment tool for family members. Each person can fill it out independently and then come together as a family unit to share the support they can provide. This identifies the caregiver's skills and strengths in different areas. This allows the individual and family to build their team of support within the family unit. As a family, you can see the gaps or areas that require more knowledge or skill building.

8.3.3 Doug and Stacy (Older Sister)

Doug is a 57-year-old gentleman with Down Syndrome who has developed dementia. His parents are deceased, and he lives in a co-housing community with his older sister Stacy (67 years old) and her husband. Before the COVID-19 pandemic, Doug went to Jazzercise, saw the horses near his house, and went to his day program twice a week. When Stacy was not able to provide transportation, someone from Jazzercise picked Doug up and he was also invited to lead part of the routine. The goal of Doug's future plan is to "make him feel comfortable because he doesn't always know he's home." Stacy has a long history of being a caregiver, first for her mother with dementia, her father with cancer, and now her younger brother Doug. In the context of her relationship with Doug, Stacy defines resilience as the following:

> I'm grateful for the things that didn't change – Doug's humor, caring for animals, love of country music. There is always a reminder of who Doug is – keeps people engaged with him. He is very much a part of life. Things we do together are part of our lives. People are saying hello and know who we are. Resilience is the capacity to stay calm and centered and face challenges and opportunities with a mindset of honoring Doug for who he is. That I am okay too. Not being too hard on myself and on Doug. Make changes on a day-to-day basis. We might not get everything done today. Find joyful times during the day.

Future Planning worksheets recommended for Doug, his family, and support providers include (1) Checklist of Daily Activities and (2) The Meaning of Hope. The checklist of daily activities can be completed at different intervals to identify changing abilities and support needs. It can be completed by formal and informal caregivers to identify the amount of supports needed. As Doug and Stacy grow older together and face the challenges of having dementia, The Meaning of Hope can help them to reframe "hope" during the last stage of life.

8.3.4 Angelo and Maria (Sister)

Angelo is a 31-year-old gentleman who has two older sisters. He is closest in age to his sister Maria who is 33. Angelo is on the autism spectrum and "he has experienced a lot in his life – discrimination, bullying and living in a society where he is constantly reminded of his limitations." Maria thinks about Angelo's future a lot.

> As they (parents) age, I think about what his life will be like, how he will fare, and what he will do to maintain happiness in his personal life. I think losing my parents one day will be a profound loss for him in ways I can't begin to describe. He follows my mother around wherever she goes. He is extremely attached to her. She (mother) had heart surgery last year and that's when I started to think about her role shifting as she ages. My father has also had cancer twice, has COPD, and a blood disorder. In these past few years, I have thought a lot about my role increasing in his life.

Maria feels her role is "being his rock." Angelo and his parents recently decided to move out of California and will be living 12 minutes away from Maria. As a sibling, she defines resilience as "helping him acknowledge and work through challenges he faces and allowing him to be the problem-solver in his own life while providing guidance and support. To give him confidence and celebrate how strong he is."

Moving to a new city and being close to family offers opportunities to learn additional skills and create a sense of belonging in new settings. The experiences individuals with IDD face in their earlier years often influence how and when families plan. It is never too early to explore what the future can look like. *Future Planning* worksheets recommended for Angelo and his family: (1) Employment and (2) Roommates. These worksheets allow individuals with IDD and families to express concerns, ask questions, identify opportunities, and practice the skills necessary to advocate for themselves. In the following section, the concepts of belonging and resilience will be discussed within the future planning process.

8.4 How to Foster Belonging and Resilience Through Future Planning

The literature on future planning reflects a dynamic and complex process. Individuals with IDD and family members may experience transitions where human bonds and relationships develop and wane. According to Carter (2016), "When purposeful and person-centered, healthy congregations strive to enable people with and without disabilities to flourish in community together" (p. 168). Table 8.1 (worksheet examples) uses Carter's dimensions of belonging as a guide to engage participants and enhance future plans for persons with IDD. A better understanding of how emotions are expressed, measured, and addressed will help us to encourage and support the sense of belonging proposed by Carter (2016). Table 8.2 represents potential ways to apply our knowledge about future planning to Carter's core principle of "belonging." These dimensions apply to both the individual with IDD and the older family caregiver as they both prepare for different transitions in their lives.

Navigating the future planning process while actively encouraging a sense of belonging among family members can help build family resilience. New models of family resilience point to the need to acknowledge the multiple influences on family resilience and how it can change over time in response to facing new risks (Henry et al., 2015). The future planning process will likely bring a sense of risk to the family as they weigh wishes alongside realities of existing resources. Parents and siblings of individuals with IDD who experienced the transition from institution to community living identify a process that is influenced by individual experiences. This is a difficult and emotional process that affects the entire family (Jones & Gallus, 2016). Caldwell et al. (2018) identified the importance of family choice or empowerment during transitions that occur over the life course. When families can exert their choices for community-based supports during transitions (i.e., changes in living situations and daily life activities), then this builds their family resilience

Table 8.2 Carter's dimensions of belonging and ways to enhance future planning

Dimensions of belonging	Questions and opportunities for individuals with IDD and families to enhance a sense of belonging in future plans
To be present	What barriers contribute to the absence of people who desire to participate in creating their plan? Recognize how attitudes influence the planning process Reexamine the balance between person-centered and family-centered planning Invite important people to the future planning process including siblings and other caregivers
To be invited	How do we determine if a person feels invited to participate in future planning? Provide opportunities to welcome and invite participation in future planning Explore how people can be included and allow them to have choices
To be welcome	How do we acknowledge the value of people's input? Acknowledge the desires, wishes, and preferences of persons with IDD Encourage participation in future planning despite a setback or negative experience Ensure that input is welcomed in all aspects of planning
To be known	How can we truly get to know the person in order to collaboratively build a meaningful plan? Remember that each plan is unique and dynamic Spend time during the planning process to share life experiences and activities that reflect who they are as individuals Ensure that during the person-centered process, the desires of the individual with IDD is honored while also considering the desires/needs of caregivers
To be accepted	How well do we know the individual? Are we including siblings and persons with disabilities in all aspects of the planning process? Listen to individual preferences and integrate them as much as possible Believe that individuals with IDD can actively participate in making independent decisions or supported decisions Hold planning meetings in locations and times that are accessible to individuals with IDD and their family members
To be supported	What supports are needed for fuller participation in planning? What supports are needed now and in the future? Include diversity of supports required by each individual with IDD – one size does not fit all Explore new opportunities and interventions and modify existing ones to meet interests Encourage self-advocacy during the person-centered planning process
To be cared for	What do people want? What social issues are important to them? What does it mean to a person "to be cared for?" Involves caring for the family caregiver as well as the individual with IDD Don't make assumptions about what a person wants or needs Recognize that perceptions vary even in families and among caregivers Find alternative ways to express that you care and are concerned Ask a lot of questions and provide opportunities to listen to each other

(continued)

Table 8.2 (continued)

Dimensions of belonging	Questions and opportunities for individuals with IDD and families to enhance a sense of belonging in future plans
To be befriended	How do we create opportunities for a variety of relationships in the future plan? What activities will allow people to spend time together? Recognize that relationships contribute to our sense of belonging in communities Plans should contain a relationship domain Remember that relationships develop over time and must be sustained
To be needed	What activities in the plan provide opportunities to be a valued member of a group or community? Respect the reciprocity between individual with IDD and their caregiver Understand that to be valued is expressed in different ways Opportunities are fluid and evolve over time so they require reevaluation on a regular basis
To be loved	How is love or being loved expressed in the future plan? What is the language of love? Ensure that individuals with IDD and caregivers are valued during the future planning process Identify what individuals need to feel loved or to express love Recognize and respect that love comes in many forms

(ability to positively adapt when facing risk situations). Likewise, individuals with IDD, parents, and siblings can make uninformed choices that lead to increased risk when information and supports are lacking, when systems have inadequate long-term services and supports, and when plans are made suddenly without an understanding of the characteristics and wishes of the person with IDD.

Considering the complexities of choice and risk faced when making decisions about the future, planning should support the empowerment of family members to have choice regarding their preferences for community-based supports and services they want or need to access. When aging family caregivers of adults with IDD engage in problem solving and finding solutions activities, they demonstrate improved resiliency and reduced caregiver burden (Piazza et al., 2014). A literature review identified both internal and external resources that contribute to resilience among individuals with IDD (Scheffers et al., 2020). The internal resources to promote resilience of individuals with IDD include providing them choice and autonomy in decisions regarding future planning preferences. For example, the individual with IDD can identify, choose, and manage the resources they need and want. External resources to build resilience involve supporting social connections and the ability to engage in fulfilling daily activities now and in the future. Individual resilience may be fostered when individuals are allowed to work through challenges they face and be recognized as the problem-solver in their own life.

Future planning, while a complex process, holds promise to build both individual and family resilience as it provides the opportunity for empowerment in responding to and planning for future life transitions. Resilience can be enhanced in future planning by using Carter's (2016) dimensions of belonging which can help facilitate open, invited, and connected decision-making. Policy and practice resources supporting future planning are included after the discussion questions in this chapter.

Resources for Individuals with IDD, Families, Service Providers, Advocates, and Professionals
Future Planning Resources

- *Future Planning: A Roadmap of Our Futures Our Wishes* is a free workbook available to guide future planning processes. https://sonoranucedd.fcm.arizona.edu/publications/OurFuturesOurWishes
- The Arc of the United States established *The Arc Center for Future Planning* to provide training and resources to individuals with IDD and their families. On *The Arc Center for Future Planning* website, there are videos, fillable forms, and state-specific future planning resources. https://futureplanning.thearc.org/pages/learn/future-planning-101
- The Future is Now is a psychoeducational intervention that consists of five 2.5 hour sessions that are co-led by peer facilitators. https://fsrtc.ahslabs.uic.edu/the-future-is-now/

Person-Centered Practice

- National Center on Advancing Person-Centered Practices and Systems (NCAPPS). Initiative from the Administration for Community Living and the Centers for Medicare & Medicaid Services. Helps states, tribes, and territories implement person-centered thinking, planning, and practice. https://ncapps.acl.gov/about-ncapps.html
- The Learning Community for Person Centered Practices. Started with the development of the essential lifestyle planning (ELP). It offers resources on person-centered thinking and ELP. https://tlcpcp.com/

Policy and Practice Resources

- The Arc of the United States and the American Association on Intellectual and Developmental Disabilities (AAIDD) collaboratively established a series of position statements which include policy and practice recommendations for quality of life, rights, life in the community, and systems of care for people with IDD. https://thearc.org/position-statements
- The University of Minnesota Institute on Community Integration publishes the *Impact* newsletter on strategies, research, and stories about the lives of individuals with disabilities. https://ici.umn.edu/series/14.
- National Resource Center for Supported-Decision Making has a resource library of both national and local resources. http://supporteddecisionmaking.org
- The ABLE National Resource Center provides information about tax-advantaged savings account that can pay for disability-related expenses. https://www.ablenrc.org/what-is-able/what-are-able-acounts/.
- Special Needs Alliance (SNA) is a national organization of attorneys who practice disability and public benefits law. The *Voice* newsletter provides

resources on a variety of topics. https://www.specialneedsalliance.org/information-center/.
- Sibling Leadership Network provides information and resources for siblings. https://siblingleadership.org/.
- The *Personal Outcome Measures® Manual for Adults* (Fourth Edition, 2017) is an interview tool that explores quality of life outcomes in multiple areas. It was developed by The Council on Quality and Leadership. https://www.c-q-l.org/resources/manuals/personal-outcome-measures-manual-for-adults/.

Questions for Thought and Discussion

1. As a provider of services and supports, what steps can be taken to encourage individuals with IDD and their caregivers to start the future planning process?
2. What part of future planning provides the most opportunity for fostering belonging?
3. What strategies can be used to incorporate the dimensions of belonging into future planning?
4. What strategies can be used to build resilience during the future planning process?

References

AARP and National Alliance for Caregiving. (2020). *Caregiving in the United States 2020.* AARP. May 2020. https://doi.org/10.26419/ppi.00103.001

Anderson, L., Hewitt, A., Pettingell, S., Lulinski, A., Taylor, M., & Reagan, J. (2018). *Family and individual needs for disability supports (v.2) community report 2017.* Research and Training Center on Community Living, Institute on Community Integration, University of Minnesota. https://ici.umn.edu/products/docs/FINDS_survey_2018.pdf

Bibby, R. (2013). 'I hope he goes first': Exploring determinants of engagement in future planning for adults with a learning disability living with ageing parents. What are the issues? A literature review. *British Journal of Learning Disabilities, 41*(2), 94–105. https://doi.org/10.1111/j.1468-3156.2012.00727.x

Botsford, A. L., & Rule, D. (2004). Evaluation of a group intervention to assist aging parents with permanency planning for an adult offspring with special needs. *Social Work, 49*(3), 423–431. https://doi.org/10.1093/sw/49.3.423

Bronfenbrenner, U. (1977). Toward an experimental ecology of human development. *American Psychologist, 32*(7), 513–531. https://doi.org/10.1037/0003-066X.32.7.513

Burke, M. M., & Heller, T. (2017). Disparities in unmet service needs among adults with intellectual and other developmental disabilities. *Journal of Applied Research in Intellectual Disabilities, 30*, 898–910. https://doi.org/10.1111/jar.12282

Burke, M., Arnold, C., & Owen, A. (2018). Identifying the correlates and barriers of future planning among parents of individuals with intellectual and developmental disabilities. *Intellectual and Developmental Disabilities, 56*(2), 90–100. https://doi.org/10.1352/1934-9556-56.2.90

Burke, M. M., Lee, C. E., Hall, S. A., & Rossetti, Z. (2019). Understanding decision making among individuals with intellectual and developmental disabilities (IDD) and their siblings. *Intellectual and Developmental Disabilities, 57*(1), 26–41. https://doi.org/10.1352/1934-9556-57.1.26

Caldwell, J. A., Jones, J. L., Gallus, K. L., & Henry, C. S. (2018). Empowerment and resilience in families of adults with intellectual and developmental disabilities. *Intellectual and Developmental Disabilities, 56*(5), 374–388. https://doi.org/10.1352/1934-9556-56.5.374

Campanella, T. M. (2015). Supported decision-making in practice. *Inclusion, 3*(1), 35–39. https://doi.org/10.1352/2326-6988-3.1.35

Carter, E. W. (2016). A place of belonging: Research at the intersection of faith and disability. *Review and Expositor, 113*, 167–180. https://doi.org/10.1177/0034637316637861

Coyle, C. E., Kramer, J., & Mutchler, J. E. (2014). Aging together: Sibling carers of adults with intellectual and developmental disabilities. *Journal of Policy and Practice in Intellectual Disabilities, 11*(4), 302–312. https://doi.org/10.1080/08959420.2015.1096142

Dillenburger, K., & McKerr, L. (2011). 'How long are we able to go on? Issues faced by older family caregivers of adults with disabilities. *British Journal of Learning Disabilities, 39*, 29–38. https://doi.org/10.1111/j.1468-3156.2010.00613.x

Dolan, E., Lane, J., Hillis, G., & Delanty, N. (2019). Changing trends in life expectancy in intellectual disability over time. *Irish Medical Journal, 112*(9), P1006. http://www.imj.ie/wp-content/uploads/2019/10/Changing-Trends-in-Life-Expectancy-in-Intellectual-Disability-Over-Time.pdf

Edelson, S. M., Nicholas, D. B., Stoddart, K. P., Bauman, M. B., Mawlam, L., Lawson, W. B., Jose, C., Morris, R., & Wright, S. D. (2021). Strategies for research, practice, and policy for autism in later life: A report from a think tank on aging and autism. *Journal of Autism and Developmental Disorders, 51*, 382–390. https://doi.org/10.1007/s10803-020-04514-3

Ervin, D. A., Hennan, B., Merrick, J., & Moran, M. (2014). Health care for persons with intellectual and developmental disability in the community. *Frontiers in Public Health, 2*(83). https://doi.org/10.3389/fpubh.2014.00083

Factor, A., Heller, T., & Janicki, M. (2012). *Bridging the aging and developmental disabilities service networks: Challenges and best practices*. Institute on Disability and Human Development, University of Illinois at Chicago. https://www.aucd.org/template/news.cfm?news_id=8557

Haley, W. E., & Perkins, E. A. (2004). Current status and future directions in family caregiving and aging people with intellectual disabilities. *Journal of Policy and Practice in Intellectual Disabilities, 1*(1), 24–30. https://doi.org/10.1111/j.1741-1130.2004.04004.x

Heller, T., & Caldwell, J. (2006). Supporting aging caregivers and adults with developmental disabilities in future planning. *Mental Retardation, 44*(3), 189–202. https://doi.org/10.1352/0047-6765(2006)44[189:SACAAW]2.0.CO;2

Heller, T., Stafford, P., Davis, L. A., Sedlezky, L., & Gaylord, V. (Eds.). (Winter 2010). *Impact: Feature Issue on Aging and People with Intellectual and Developmental Disabilities, 23*(1). Institute on Community Integration, University of Minnesota and Research and Training Center on Community Living. Integration. https://publications.ici.umn.edu/impact/23-1/from-the-editors

Henry, C. S., Morris, A. S., & Harrist, A. W. (2015). Family resilience: Moving into the third wave. *Family Relations, 64*(1), 22–43. https://doi.org/10.1111/fare.12106

Hewitt, A., Lightfoot, E., Bogenschutz, M., McCormick, K., Sedlezky, L., & Doljanac, R. (2010). Parental caregivers' desires for lifetime assistance planning for future supports for their children with intellectual and developmental disabilities. *Journal of Family Social Work, 13*(5), 420–434. https://doi.org/10.1080/10522158.2010.514678

Hewitt, A., Agosta, J., Heller, T., Williamson, A. C., & Reinke, J. (2013). Families of individuals with intellectual and developmental disabilities: Policy, funding, services, and experiences. *Intellectual and Developmental Disabilities, 51*(5), 349–359. https://doi.org/10.1352/1934-9556-51.5.349

Jones, J. L., & Gallus, K. L. (2016). Understanding deinstitutionalization: What families value and desire in the transition to community living. *Research and Practice for Persons with Severe Disabilities, 41*(2), 116–131. https://doi.org/10.1177/1540796916637050

Lakin, K. C., & Burke, M. M. (2019). Looking forward: Research to respond to a rapidly aging population. *Research and Practice for Persons with Severe Disabilities, 44*(4), 280–292. https://doi.org/10.1177/1540796919882356

Lee, C., & Burke, M. M. (2020). Future planning among families of individuals with intellectual and developmental disabilities: A systematic review. *Journal of Policy and Practice in Intellectual Disabilities, 17*(2), 94–107. https://doi.org/10.1111/jppi.12324

Lee, C., Burke, M., Arnold, C. K., & Owen, A. (2019a). Correlates of current caregiving among siblings of adults with intellectual and developmental disabilities. *Journal of Applied Research in Intellectual Disabilities, 32*(6), 1490–1500. https://doi.org/10.1111/jar.12644

Lee, C., Burke, M. M., & Stelter, C. R. (2019b). Exploring the perspectives of parents and siblings toward future planning for individuals with intellectual and developmental disabilities. *Intellectual and Developmental Disabilities, 57*(3), 198–211. https://doi.org/10.1352/1934-9556-57.3.198

Lindahl, J., Stollon, N., Wu, K., Liang, A., Changolkar, S., Steinway, C., Trachtenberg, S., Coccia, A., Devaney, M., & Jan, S. (2019). Domains of planning for future long-term care of adults with intellectual and developmental disabilities: Parent and sibling perspectives. *Journal of Applied Research in Intellectual Disabilities, 32*(5), 1103–1115. https://doi.org/10.1111/jar.12600

Magaña, S., Parish, S., Morales, M. A., Li, H., & Fujiura, G. (2016). Racial and ethnic health disparities among people with intellectual and developmental disabilities. *Intellectual and Developmental Disabilities, 54*(3), 161–172. https://doi.org/10.1352/1934-9556-54.3.161

McCausland, D., Brennan, D., McCallion, P., & McCarron, M. (2019). Balancing personal wishes and caring capacity in future planning for adults with an intellectual disability living with family carers. *Journal of Intellectual Disabilities, 23*(3), 413–431. https://doi.org/10.1177/1744629519872658

Namkung, E. H., Greenberg, J. S., Mailick, M. R., & Floyd, F. J. (2018). Lifelong parenting of adults with developmental disabilities: Growth trends over 20 years in midlife and later life. *American Journal on Intellectual and Developmental Disabilities, 123*(3), 228–240. https://doi.org/10.1352/1944-7558-123.3.228

National Academies of Sciences, Engineering, and Medicine. (2018). *People living with disabilities: Health equity, health disparities, and health literacy: Proceedings of a workshop*. The National Academies Press. https://doi.org/10.17226/24741

National Quality Forum. (2020). *Person-centered planning and practice: Final report*. http://www.qualityforum.org/Publications/2020/07/Person_Centered_Planning_and_Practice_Final_Report.aspx

National Resource Center for Supported Decision-Making. (n.d.). http://www.supporteddecisionmaking.org/

Owen, A., Stober, K., Crabb, C., Mahar, E., & Heller, T. (2020). Training professionals to facilitate future planning for aging caregivers: Exploratory results from a multistate intervention. *Journal of Policy and Practice in Intellectual Disabilities*. https://doi.org/10.1111/jppi.12362

Perkins, E. A., & Haley, W. E. (2013). Emotional and tangible reciprocity in middle-and older-aged carers of adult with intellectual disabilities. *Journal of Policy and Practice in Intellectual Disabilities, 10*(4), 334–344. https://doi.org/10.1111/jppi.12061

Piazza, V. E., Floyd, F. J., Mailick, M. R., & Greenberg, J. S. (2014). Coping and psychological health of aging parents of adult children with developmental disabilities. *American Journal on Intellectual and Developmental Disabilities, 119*(2), 186–198. https://doi.org/10.1352/1944-7558-119.2.186

Rossetti, Z., Stanisz, H. D., & Kramer, J. (2020). Siblings of people with IDD: The adult years. In V. D. Gaylord & J. K. Stewart (Managing Eds.) and K. Arnold, E. Holl, E. S. Tanis, S. Hall, & J. W. Smith (Eds.), *Impact: Feature Issue on Siblings of People with Intellectual, Developmental, and Other Disabilities, 32*(2). Institute on Community Integration, University of Minnesota & Research Training Center on Community Living. https://publications.ici.umn.edu/impact/32-2/siblings-of-people-with-idd-the-adult-years

Ryan, A., Taggart, L., Truesdale-Kennedy, M., & Slevin, E. (2014). Issues in caregiving for older people with intellectual disabilities and their ageing family carers: A review and commentary. *International Journal of Older People Nursing, 9*(3), 217–226. https://doi.org/10.1111/opn.12021

Scheffers, F., van Vugt, E., & Moonen, X. (2020). Resilience in the face of adversity in adults with an intellectual disability: A literature review. *Journal of Applied Research in Intellectual Disabilities*. https://doi.org/10.1111/jar.12720

Schepens, H. R. M. M., Van Puyenbroeck, J., & Maes, B. (2019). How to improve the quality of life of elderly people with intellectual disability: A systematic literature review of support strategies. *Journal of Applied Research in Intellectual Disabilities, 32*(3), 483–521. https://doi.org/10.1111/jar.12559

Scott, H. M., & Havercamp, S. M. (2014). Race and health disparities in adults with intellectual and developmental disabilities living in the United States. *Intellectual and Developmental Disabilities, 52*(6), 409–418. https://doi.org/10.1352/1934-9556-52.6.409

Shogren, K. A., & Wehmeyer, M. L. (2015). A framework for research and intervention design in supported decision-making. *Inclusion, 3*(1), 17–23. https://doi.org/10.1352/2326-6988-3.1.17

Shogren, K., Wehmeyer, M., Lassmann, H., & Forber-Pratt, A. (2017). Supported decision making: A synthesis of the literature across intellectual disability, mental health, and aging. *Education and Training in Autism and Developmental Disabilities, 52*(2), 144–157. https://doi.org/10.2307/26420386

Smith, G. C., Majeski, R. A., & McClenny, B. (1996). Psychoeducational support groups for aging parents: Development and preliminary outcomes. *Mental Retardation, 34*(3), 172–181.

Tanis, E. S., Lulinski, A., Wu, J., Braddock, D., & Hemp, R. (2020). *The state of the states in intellectual and developmental disabilities*. University of Colorado. www.stateofthestates.org

Tencza, M., & Forsythe, L. (2019). Transition-of-care planning: Preparing for the future care of the individual with intellectual and developmental disabilities. *Journal of Intellectual Disabilities*. https://doi.org/10.1177/1744629519883453. Advance online publication.

The Arc. (2018). *Position statements*. https://thearc.org/wp-content/uploads/2019/08/18-126-Position-Statement-Update_v4-1.pdf

The Arc Center for Future Planning. (n.d.). *Future planning, 101*. https://futureplanning.thearc.org/pages/learn/future-planning-101

Tomasa, L. (2018). *Future planning: A roadmap of our futures our wishes*. Sonoran Center for Excellence in Disabilities. https://sonoranucedd.fcm.arizona.edu/publications/OurFuturesOurWishes

Tomasa, L., & Shirai, Y. (2008). Aging and transitions project: Technical report and white paper. [Unpublished report]. Sonoran Center for Excellence in Disabilities, University of Arizona. https://sonoranucedd.fcm.arizona.edu/publications/169

U.S. Department of Health and Human Services (USDHHS). (2005). *The Surgeon General's call to action to improve the health and wellness of people with disabilities*. U.S. Department of Health and Human Services, Office of the Surgeon General. https://www.ncbi.nlm.nih.gov/books/NBK44667/

Vespa, J., Medina, L., & Armstrong, D. M. (Issued 2018, Revised 2020). *Demographic turning points for the United States: Population projections for 2020 to 2060*, Current Population Reports, P25-1144, U.S. Census Bureau. https://www.census.gov/content/dam/Census/library/publications/2020/demo/p25-1144.pdf

Walker, R., & Hutchinson, C. (2018). Planning for the future among older parents of adult offspring with intellectual disability living at home and in the community: A systematic review of qualitative studies. *Journal of Intellectual & Developmental Disability, 43*(4), 453–462. https://doi.org/10.3109/13668250.2017.1310823

Whitlatch, M., & Ullman, S. (2020). *Debunking the myths of supported decision-making and guardianship* [webinar Sept 7]. The Arc Center for Future Planning. https://futureplanning.thearc.org/pages/learn/where-to-start/webinars/archived-webinars

Williamson, H. J., & Perkins, E. A. (2014). Family caregivers of adults with intellectual and developmental disabilities: Outcomes associated with U.S. services and supports. *Intellectual and Developmental Disabilities, 52*(2), 147–159. https://doi.org/10.1352/1934-9556-52.2.147

Yamaki, K., Hsieh, K., & Heller, T. (2009). Health profile of aging family caregivers supporting adults with intellectual and developmental disabilities at home. *Intellectual and Developmental Disabilities, 47*(6), 425–435. https://doi.org/10.1352/1934-9556-47.6.425

Epilogue

Jennifer L. Jones and Kami L. Gallus

We are so grateful for the opportunity to work alongside the many thoughtful and passionate authors in this volume. The insights provided by this distinguished group of scholars shine the light on present pathways to fostering resilient families and communities where individuals with intellectual and developmental disabilities (IDD) experience true belonging and an enhanced quality of life. The work of these authors alongside self-advocates, family members, and professionals is transforming our scholarship and our communities such that our once held hope for belonging is becoming reality. Throughout the pages of this book, we were reminded again and again that for all of us relationships are at the heart of who we are and who we are becoming. *The need to belong is universal* and key to fostering individual, family, and community resilience.

As we embarked on the journey of writing this volume, we had the opportunity to gather as colleagues, authors, and professionals. Across the two-day Chautauqua conference on family resilience in March 2020, we shared how our individual work creates belonging for individuals with IDD and their families. When we gathered for dinner, I (JJ) asked my dear friend and colleague, Ann Turnbull, to share a story she had told me years before. With her permission, we are closing this volume with her powerful story of how belonging improves our lives and builds resilient families and communities.

J. L. Jones · K. L. Gallus
Human Development and Family Science, Oklahoma State University, Stillwater, OK, USA
e-mail: Jennifer.jones@okstate.edu; kami.gallus@okstate.edu

J. L. Jones, K. L. Gallus (eds.), *Belonging and Resilience in Individuals with Developmental Disabilities*, Emerging Issues in Family and Individual Resilience, https://doi.org/10.1007/978-3-030-81277-5

The Green Card of Friendship: A Short Story by Ann Turnbull

My son, Jay, was a pioneer of supported living in the late 1980s. The only options for people with highly intensive support needs in our community were group homes and sheltered workshops. Jay started in these segregated programs, with the vision of his Dad (Rud) and I being that we would devote ourselves to intensive advocacy to transform this disability-only system and replace it with supported employment and supported living. Sadly, we found the interest of program leaders for transformation sorely lacking. Jay engaged in his own advocacy for inclusive living through aggressive and oppositional behavior that resulted in his expulsion from a group home within just a couple of months of his entry. Rud and I were told by the professional staff that one of the big problems for Jay was that we were highly "unrealistic" about the extent and impact of his multiple disabilities (i.e., intellectual disability, autism, bipolar disorder). They told us repeatedly that Jay was "far too disabled" to function successfully in the group home and workshop. They implied that a more restrictive setting such as an institutional placement would likely be more appropriate.

Rud and I swore that would never happen. We set out to develop supported employment and supported living for him and other adults with intense support needs in our community. We set up an "action team" comprised of family and friends to help us create a full vision of inclusive living and to put that vision into place—step by step—until all of those small steps accumulated and morphed into Jay's whole life.

There came a time when the priority for the action team was taking a next step for Jay to learn to use public transportation, and the place to start was independently using taxis. There were several reasons why I was especially scared for Jay to use a taxi because, as much as I value looking on the positive side of everything, I thought about the possibility that the taxi driver might bully him or steal his money. I even thought of the worst-case scenario of the driver taking him to a secluded place and molesting him. I hated to think any of these bad things could possibly happen; but what if one or more did happen to Jay? The prospects generated huge fear and hesitancy in moving ahead. Our action team was more optimistic than I was. They encouraged—really insisted—that I should go to the local taxi company and see what kind of supports we might be able to figure out to address these potential challenges.

I didn't know what to say to the owners of the local taxi company, and I didn't want to accuse them of unethical or dangerous behavior. I felt very ill-at-ease driving into the dirt parking lot of the trailer on the edge of town where the taxi company had their office. Not knowing what in the world I was going to say, I went inside the trailer and met the owner, Shirley, who was sitting at a dilapidated desk dispatching with her drivers. It was like a scene from a 1950s movie.

I introduced myself and started rambling in telling her about Jay, the life he wanted for himself in the community, and his intensive support needs associated with his multiple disabilities. Shirley was nodding and conveying empathy as I sheepishly told her about my worries. I felt so ashamed of having these fears, and I did not want in any way to insult Shirley and demonstrate bias toward her and her drivers. Her empathetic listening conveyed to me that she understood what I was saying. I felt as if I was engaging with a seasoned therapist who excelled in unconditional acceptance. She nodded and affirmed what I was sharing, "I understand, Ann, and if I were Jay's mother I would feel that same way. Tell me more about your worries. What else is on your mind?" I told her about bullying, and then I told her about stealing. I finally got up the courage to tell her about my worry concerning someone molesting Jay.

When I was done and feeling foolish, she reached across her desk to embrace me. She then opened her rickety desk drawer and pulled out two crinkled pieces of construction paper, a red one and green one. She said, "I'm giving you my green card of friendship. I'm giving you my green card of problem solving. I'm giving you my green card of caring about your son." Tears rolled down my face. I was at a loss for words. I could not believe I was in a trailer of a taxi company, and I was getting this kind of absolute support of my heartfelt worries and supreme offer of friendship and help. I was having a hard time taking it all in so I asked, "Shirley, what do you mean?" and she said, "Ann, many of you in the University don't realize that people like me want to give back, and we want to make a difference in the lives of people. Every morning I wake up, and I ask the good Lord to let me take as many red cards as possible. You've given me your red card of worry and your red card of fear. I give you my green cards."

After exchanging cards, Shirley went on to explain how she was going to take care of each of my concerns. She said she would be on the dispatcher with the driver from the time Jay got in the taxi until the time he got out. She could give me her solemn vow that Jay would be safe and treated with respect. Shirley then described that she had 22 drivers, and she had never matched a rider with driver, but she would match Jay with just 1 driver so they could develop a friendship and trust each other. She said "I don't want to limit your son, so I'll bring in another driver when the time is right and then another until he rides with all 22. Let me think overnight about which driver should go first."

Shirley called me the next day and described how she had picked Jim to be the first driver and had told Jim all about our conversation. She shared that Jim's only question was this: "Shirley, why did you pick me?" Laughingly, Shirley said she responded by saying, "Jim, you need a friend as much as Jay Turnbull needs one!" I learned a profound lesson from Shirley. It is this: Outside of the disability world, as well as outside of one's family and friendship network, there are thousands of extraordinary people who have green cards to share. As we strive to advance belonging for individuals with disabilities and their families, a priority goal should be to nurture relationships and expand exponentially the red cards that are taken in and the green cards that are boundlessly shared.

Index

J. L. Jones, K. L. Gallus (eds.), *Belonging and Resilience in Individuals with Developmental Disabilities*, Emerging Issues in Family and Individual Resilience, https://doi.org/10.1007/978-3-030-81277-5

The manufacturer's authorised representative in the EU is Springer Nature Customer Service Centre GmbH, Europaplatz 3, 69115 Heidelberg, Germany. If you have any concerns regarding our products, please contact ProductSafety@springernature.com

Printed and bound by CPI Group (UK) Ltd, Croydon, CR0 4YY
28/09/2026
02224086-0018